Life with Chronic Illness

Life with Chronic Illness
Social and Psychological Dimensions

Ariela Royer

PRAEGER

Westport, Connecticut
London

Library of Congress Cataloging-in-Publication Data

Royer, Ariela.
   Life with chronic illness : social and psychological dimensions /
Ariela Royer.
     p. cm.
   Includes bibliographical references and index.
   ISBN 0-275-96123-0 (alk. paper)
    1. Chronic diseases—Social aspects. 2. Chronic diseases—
Psychological aspects. I. Title.
   RA644.5.R69   1998
   616′.001′9—DC21   98-11133

British Library Cataloguing in Publication Data is available.

Library of Congress Catalog Card Number: 98-11133
ISBN: 0-275-96123-0

First published in 1998

Praeger Publishers, 88 Post Road West, Westport, CT 06881
An imprint of Greenwood Publishing Group, Inc.

Printed in the United States of America

The paper used in this book complies with the
Permanent Paper Standard issued by the National
Information Standards Organization (Z39.48–1984).

10 9 8 7 6 5 4 3 2

I dedicate this book to my mother Sabina Ronis Benzion and to my mentor Rue Marie Bucher. Unfortunately these two women knew only too well what it means to live with chronic illness. My greatest debt, however, is to all the wonderful men and women who so generously shared with me their experiences, their wisdom and the stories of their lives.

Contents

Preface

When people become ill, the physical symptoms and medical aspects are the first and most important concerns that have to be dealt with. However, once symptoms are diagnosed, brought under control, acute crises averted, and necessary medical regimens established, other concerns related to living with long-term illness emerge as important concerns to the sufferers. Concerns arise such as: Am I going to be able to keep my job?; How am I going to pay my medical bills, or any of my bills, for that matter?; What will happen to my marriage, or to my relationships?; Will I be able to participate in valued social activities?; and other similar concerns, as expressed by all the people I interviewed.

This book was conceived out of my interest in the study of health and illness, particularly of illness behavior. Specifically, I wanted to explore what it is like to have a chronic—that is, long-term—and incurable illness in our society and how people experience and attempt to control such an illness in their everyday lives. Thus, the general question that guided my research was, What is it like to live with a long-term chronic illness in this society? I had other questions as well: How do chronically ill persons define, explain, and attribute their illness? How do they learn to interpret and assess changes in their condition? What kinds of efforts (successful or unsuccessful) do they make to maintain some control over and keep ahead of their illness? And what effects does their illness itself have on these interpretive processes?

I focused on these questions in an effort to examine how people adapt to and normalize their lives with an ongoing illness. In fact, I was mostly interested in finding people who were successful in dealing with the impact of chronic illness on their lives, in the hope of learning from their experiences.

Thus, the model for my book draws heavily on the sociological perspectives of symbolic interactionism (Blumer 1969), phenomenology (Schutz 1971), and ethnomethodology (Cicourel 1974; Dreitzel 1970; Garfinkel 1967; Psathas 1973; Sudnow 1972). Symbolic interactionism was the first sociological perspective to seriously consider social meanings as the essence of everyday-life sociology. As Blumer (1969, p.183) suggests, an individual's behavior "is not a result of such things as environmental pressures, stimuli, motives, attitudes and ideas, but arises instead from how he interprets and handles these things in the action which he is constructing." According to these perspectives, people interpret their own and each other's actions, and on the basis of these interpretations, decide which course of action to employ. The self is crucially important in determining the interpretation and resulting actions that occur.

For instance, when people get sick and visit a doctor, they do not immediately stop thinking or behaving the way they normally do. Thinking takes place in contexts of feeling, prior experience and learning. People learn to make decisions long before they come to a doctor's office. They learn at home, at school, at work, and at play. There they learn to make decisions that "feel right" to them. Whether those decisions are right or are being made in a rational way is another matter. There are indications, for instance, that even people who are capable of thinking rationally most of the time tend to fall back on regressive patterns of thought and behavior when experiencing the pain and fear that accompany illness or injury. Indeed, there might be many reasons why people are sometimes afraid to be rational even when they have the capacity to be, as well as reasons why people often are not capable of being rational even when they are not conscious of fear. On the other hand, what appear as irrational and regressive patterns of thought and behavior to health care professionals and family caregivers are actually, in many cases, rational normalization tactics from the point of view of chronically ill persons.

The main point is that when people are seriously ill and/or in pain, they seek explanations for what causes their suffering. The explanations and behaviors that are right at hand are those that people learn throughout their lives, and we, in turn, can learn much about people in general by tapping into these processes.

Early in my study, I drew on the insight and experience of Professor R. Bucher, who herself was dealing with many of the problems discussed. I also drew on my own past experiences with chronic conditions. My mother fell ill with arteriosclerosis and suffered for 10 years before she died at the age of 59. For reasons I do not recall now, it was decided that she could not be moved to a hospital and had to remain confined to her bed, for at least a whole month, during the initial acute episode of the illness. The doctor who was treating her made one house call a day and gave me a crash course in the art of nursing a patient, including how to give her the needed daily injections. My father, according to the prevailing gender role norms of the times, was not expected to take on this responsibility. So, out of necessity, at the age of 18, for all practical purposes I became a nurse! I was also expected to fulfill my mother's household duties while she was unable to do so. Thus, with the help of my 12-year-old sister, both of us managed as well as we could. More than four decades later, I still remember the high level of anxiety I experienced, not only because my mother could have died at the time, but because she could have died as a consequence of my inadequacy. Unfortunately, this was not my only experience with chronic illness. At the time of my mother's illness, between the ages of 12 and 21, I myself suffered from a chronic illness, asthma, which at times made my life unbearable. Although severely debilitated, I tried most of the time to function as though everything was "normal." In retrospect, I recognize that I used many of the normalization strategies discussed in Part III of this book. In fact, because of my own experiences with chronic illness, as both a sufferer and a caregiver, I was sensitized to the many normalization tactics people use. Many of these normalization tactics are generally perceived by caregivers as well as health care professionals as maladaptive behaviors non-compliant with traditional medical advice rather than "survival tactics" for chronically ill people.

In fact, healthy persons may have no idea what it feels like to experience a particular chronic illness or disability, or to care for someone who has that experience. Even health care professionals, doctors and nurses, who are knowledgeable about the medical and nursing facts of the situation, may know little about individual responses to the illness experience, the symptoms or reactions with which a particular patient and family have to cope, or the resources available to assist recovery or adaptation.

There have been an increasing number of studies in the last three decades on adaptation to chronic conditions (Gussow 1964; Kasl and Cobb 1964; Kemp and Vash 1971; Fishman and Schneider 1972; Mechanic 1972; Feldman 1974; Hyman 1975; Barsky 1976; Locker 1983; Schneider and Conrad 1983; Strauss et al. 1984; Corbin and Strauss 1988; Charmaz 1991), which indicate that how well people manage their chronic conditions is associated more with psychosocial factors than the strictly medical diagnosis of their physical problems would suggest. In particular, we have learned quite a bit about the way people construct adaptations to the problems of living with specific conditions such as arthritis (Moos 1964, 1965; Markson 1971; Wiener 1975), heart disease (Lewis 1966; Croog 1981), epilepsy (Bagley 1971; West 1970b, 1979b; Oliver 1980; Schneider and Conrad 1983), and multiple sclerosis (Davis 1973; Braham et al. 1975).

Many social scientific studies have examined various aspects of illness experience, including doctor-patient relations, peoples' experiences with hospital stays, and coping with the problems of a particular illness. Although insightful and useful, because they reveal important aspects of the illness experience, these studies do not give us the whole picture of everyday existence in the life of a chronically ill person because most of these studies have been done by health care professionals from a medical point of view, mainly dealing with the physical symptoms and medical aspects of an illness—but for the most part ignoring or minimizing other concerns also central to people suffering from long-term chronic illness.

With some notable exceptions (Strauss 1975; Schneider and Conrad 1983; Strauss et al. 1984; Corbin and Strauss 1988), most studies, even those attempting to examine illness experience, are studies of "patienthood." It is true, of course, that part of being ill often does include being a patient, though only a small amount of time is spent by most sick people in hospitals and in direct interaction with doctors and/or other health care professionals. Furthermore, patienthood in these studies, if examined, focuses mainly on the staff's view of patients, for the most part ignoring how such care providers and contexts are perceived and experienced by patients themselves. Indeed, being a patient and/or being in a hospital represents only a small part of the total experience of coping with everyday aspects of an ongoing illness. Understandably, these aspects are largely invisible to health care professionals and outside of their responsibilities to patients, yet these concerns are of crucial importance to chronically ill persons and their families.

Similarly, illness behavior studies often use concepts such as "health beliefs" or "sick role," or construct other analytic categories that give short shrift to the experience of illness itself (e.g., Robinson 1971). While the experience of illness typically does begin before one becomes a patient and does include patients' perceptions of their medical treatment (Zola 1973), these studies typically frame the experience of illness in terms of the perception of and reaction to symptoms, social networks used in locating help (Freidson 1960), and the decision to seek medical care (Stimson and Webb 1975). The illness experience itself is a secondary concern even in studies on "illness careers" (Suchman 1965a, 1965b). These studies draw attention more to the patient vis-à-vis health providers and/or institutional contexts than to how such providers and contexts are perceived and experienced by the patient. These perceptions are important resources on which chronically ill persons rely to inform and guide their conduct during their illnesses.

My purpose in this discussion is not to criticize these important studies but to show the necessity of a study like this one also, in presenting a more realistic understanding of the total experience of living with an ongoing illness. Since most of the daily management of chronic illness actually takes place in the home and is performed by ill persons themselves, it is crucial to take into consideration their experiences and perceptions of the situation together with those of health care professionals.

Lincoln and Guba (1985, p. 83) note that

a perception (à la blind men and the elephant) is a partial, incomplete view of something that is nevertheless real, and capable of different interpretation when seen from different viewpoints. It is partial and incomplete only because each perception yields experience of only a limited number of parts of the whole (the tail, the trunk, the leg, and so on). . . . Reality for any individual – or group or even discipline – is at best only a partial picture of the whole, and will continue to remain so. But both the naive (or hypothetical) realists and the perceptual realists adopt the ontological position that there is a reality out there, a "real" reality, if you will; the differences lie between what the two groups believe is knowable about that reality.

These researchers, who advocate the naturalistic paradigm, also add, "with a sufficient body of research into the physical, social, and temporal, reality should rise out of the mists that enshroud it and become known."

Corbin and Strauss (1988, pp. xi–xii) in *Unending Work and Care: Managing Chronic Illness at Home,* take a similar point of view for practical purposes, since they are also concerned with finding ways to help chronically ill people manage their illness more effectively. In the preface of their book, they state that

policy planning and decisions about managing chronic illness are sometimes unrealistic and, therefore, ineffective, because they are developed by people whose experiences and perspectives are far removed from those of the chronically ill and their families. The principal field of battle lies in the homes of the chronically ill, so the more we know about what happens there, the better our policies can be.

Indeed, the category of chronic conditions is far from homogeneous, but the various conditions exert, by definition, some long-term influence upon the lives of sufferers. On the surface these illnesses seem to be very different from each other. The ways they impact the sufferers and their families, however, are very similar.

At the present time, as there are millions of people in our society afflicted to various degrees by many chronic conditions, we ought to recognize the difficulties they encounter in their daily lives and find means of helping them function in ways acceptable to themselves. The first steps in that direction are to identify the most problematic aspects of living with chronic conditions and to describe the strategies chronically ill people use to overcome these difficulties. Thus, we might find ways to help them lead relatively normal and productive lives. That is the main purpose of my book.

Acknowledgments

Acknowledging my indebtedness is exceedingly difficult. No one knows fully the experiences and people that have shaped her or his thinking. I found the insights in Goffman's, Friedson's, Zola's and Strauss' works to be particularly significant. I am indebted to Rue Bucher and Steve Warner both for teaching me critical thinking and for their years of help and guidance, I am especially grateful.

I owe thanks in many directions. First of all, thanks to all those people and experiences that enabled me to get to "this place" in my life. Thanks to my friends and colleagues in the Department of Sociology at Indiana University South Bend, especially to Mike Keen and Scott Sernau, who supplied support and encouragement that has been very much appreciated.

Many thanks to Lynn Taylor, Christina Lester, and Heidi Straight for their unstinting editorial efforts, for their patience, and terrific support.

Above all, plain thanks to my wonderful children Lydia, Bryan, Christina, and their equally wonderful significant others, Kenny, Kristen, and Greg; to my younger but wiser sister Hannah, and her family Alan, Mark and Amy; to my magnificient grandchildren Eryn, Anna, and brand new baby Wynne. There are three dedicated hard working physicians, and a physical therapist among them, I appreciate and respect their work very much. For my family's love and encouragement, all these years, my deepest gratitude.

Introduction

Chronic Illness: An Overview

What we do to the physically handicapped and chronically ill is what we do to ourselves.

—Irving K. Zola

Long-term chronic illness, be it physical or mental, is catastrophic, and even with much-improved treatment and preventive methods, it is here to stay. It will not disappear, despite the many marvelous advances in medical knowledge and technology, many of which prolong life but tend to create certain new problems in living for the individuals involved.

The term "chronic illness" refers to those disease categories for which there is no known "cure," to conditions that are ineradicable and usually progressive. The Commission on Chronic Illness (1956, p. 1) defines chronic illness as "all impairments or deviations from normal which have one or more of the following characteristics: are permanent, leave residual disability, are caused by non-reversible pathological alteration, require special training of the patient for rehabilitation, and/or may be expected to require a long period of supervision, observation or care."

Physical pain, discomfort, and the effects of treatment procedures all cause the chronically ill to suffer as they experience their illness, partially because the course of illness and treatment of a chronic illness is quite different from that of an acute illness. Chronic illness often seems to begin abruptly, and sometimes insidiously, and the course of illness is long and unpredictable. Many chronic illnesses and disabling conditions are characterized by an indefinitely long plateau rather than rapidly progressive deterioration.

Although not all conditions are fatal or even terribly disabling, many are. Many have onsets fairly early in life, and affect a significant proportion of our population. Arthritis, diabetes, multiple sclerosis, stroke, cardiac incapacity, paraplegia, renal disease, some forms of cancer, and progressive blindness are a few well-known common examples. These constitute the prevalent illnesses that bring people to the doctor's office, to the emergency clinic, and into the hospital. The medical response to such conditions can usually be described as management rather than treatment of the disease itself. In fact, according to Cogswell and Weir (1973), although chronic diseases vary in course of disease and type of treatment, the total array can be considered a single category on the basis of two similarities: (1) the patient is an active participant in her or his medical care; and (2) the goal of treatment is control, or management, since "recovery" at this stage of medical knowledge is usually impossible.

Furthermore, chronic illnesses are characterized by long-term progressive courses, relatively unpredictable remissions and exacerbations, and disabling effects. They are also frequently accompanied by minimally effective treatments despite large efforts at palliation, by social stigma, and by isolation, with some degree of dependency augmented by a lack of a legitimate cultural role and shared definitions. Consequently, they create social and treatment ambiguities at the very least. They also often create conflicts of interpretation among patients and health care workers, significant others, and funding agencies. Chronic illnesses, then, are disproportionately intrusive upon the lives of the ill and their families, as well as expensive to treat and manage.

Thus the crises brought on by chronic illnesses certainly result in an imbalance or disorganization of body, mind, and spirit. Although each person may react differently to the crises, everyone experiences such imbalance and disharmony, and this can turn individuals either inward and toward or away from a personal growth process. For some, the illness provides the first opportunity to confront their own dependency, vulnerability, and mortality. For others, it leads to great changes in their priorities and to a renewed sense of urgency to leave a legacy of accomplishments. Paradoxically, then, the chronic illness becomes a spiritual encounter as well as a physical and emotional experience.

In sum, chronic illness refers to an altered health state that will not be cured by a simple surgical procedure or a short course of medical therapy. Although each chronic illness presents some unique demands on the patient and family, two generalizations can be made about the consequences of chronic illnesses: (1) the person with a chronic illness experiences impaired functioning in more than one, often multiple, body, mind, and spirit systems; (2) the illness-related demands on the individual are never completely eliminated.

PREVALENCE OF CHRONIC ILLNESS

Long-term chronic illness is a new phenomenon in the history of the world. Prior to the twentieth century, illness was generally acute and limited in duration, and it was usually fatal. Many common chronic illnesses such as arthritis and diabetes probably existed also, but since technology to keep these people alive for long periods of time was not as well developed, most of these people died from an acute episode of their illness (e.g., diabetic coma) soon after the onset of their illness. According to McKinlay and McKinlay (1990):

In 1900, about 40 percent of all deaths were accounted for by eleven major infectious diseases, 16 percent by three chronic conditions [heart disease, cancer, and stroke], 4 percent by accidents, and the remainder (37 percent) by all other causes. By 1973, only 6 percent of all deaths were due to these eleven infectious diseases, 58 percent to the same three chronic conditions, 9 percent to accidents, and 27 percent were contributed by other causes. (p. 15)

Advances in sanitation, refrigeration, living conditions, and personal hygiene, as well as breakthroughs in the biological sciences in terms of antibiotics and vaccines and other advances in medical knowledge, have resulted in impressive gains in our society over infectious and parasitic diseases. These gains, however, have not been entirely free of problematic consequences. Technologies for successful treatment or prevention of acute life-threatening illnesses have resulted in an increase in the numbers of individuals with residual limitations and chronic physical or emotional problems that continue long after the acute stage of the illness has been successfully managed.

Whereas mortality from infectious diseases steadily declined after 1900, the proportion of deaths from major chronic diseases such as heart disease, cancer, and stroke increased more than 250 percent (U.S. DHEW 1979), and these conditions are presently the three major causes of death in the United States (U.S. DHHS 1981). These three conditions alone account for 20 percent of physician visits, 40 percent of hospital days, 50 percent of bed disability days, and eventually 75 percent of all deaths (Senate Special Committee on Aging 1985). Other significant conditions, such as arthritis, diabetes, renal failure, and mental illness, are also leading health problems in the United States, and even though they are not directly reflected in mortality statistics, they provoke considerable sickness disability, damage to self-identity, and economic loss.

Mortality statistics do not reflect the amount of morbidity present in a society; in other words, just because people live longer does not mean that they are healthier. For example, in our society, arthritis in its various forms afflicts 37 million people (Lawrence et. al. 1989); 11 million persons suffer from diabetes (American Diabetes Association 1986); five million have had cancer (American Cancer Society 1989); almost another five million have a history of heart attack and/or chest pain; and more than two million individuals have sustained a stroke (American Heart Association 1988). Nearly 29 million suffer from hypertension (U.S. Bureau of the Census 1987); and estimates of the prevalence of high blood pressure run as high as 60 million people (American Heart Association 1988). There might be some overlap in these statistics, because many people suffer from more than one chronic condition.

Antonovsky (1979) estimated that 54 percent of the American population has at least one chronic condition, and this statistic has not changed significantly in the last 18 years. At any given time, 50 percent of our population has some chronic condition that requires medical management. A more startling statistic is that most of us will eventually develop at least one chronic illness or disability that may ultimately be the cause of our death.

Furthermore, in spite of a popular belief linking chronic illness mainly to aging, most chronic problems extend across the life span. Babies saved in sophisticated intensive care nurseries often develop disabilities and systemic illnesses (some not known until later) that are incurable and have to be dealt with throughout their lives. One of every seven men and one of every eight women between the ages of 17 and 44 are limited in their major activity—the ability to work, keep house, or go to school—because of a chronic condition. At ages 65 and over, nearly three-fifths of men and two-fifths of women are so handicapped. Cole (1979) stated that "the increased prevalence rate of chronic conditions with advance in age is striking. More than 50 percent of persons of both sexes in the 17–44 age group are afflicted, as are about 70 percent of persons aged 45–64, and about 85 percent of persons aged 65 and over" (Cole 1979, p. 38).

According to the U.S. Bureau of the Census (1986), in actual numbers, approximately 110 million people, almost 50 percent of the American population, have one or more chronic health condition. Of the persons afflicted, nearly 32.4 million people are limited in their normal daily activities as a result of their illness. Out of these 32.4 million persons, approximately 11 million are under the age of 45 years, 11 million are 45 to 64 years of age, and 10.3 million are 65 years of age and older. Even if the proportion of people with chronic illness is assumed to remain constant, absolute numbers in the population will increase as a consequence of the aging population.

All these statistics might seem confusing because the exact numbers of people affected by chronic illness are difficult to assess. Prevalence studies produce variable results due to the problems of both definition and measurement; these studies rely on health care utilization statistics, which do not reflect sizable segments of the population in which sufferers rarely seek "formal" health care for either religious (e.g., in the case of Christian Scientists), legal (e.g., in the case of illegal immigrants), or financial reasons. At present, it is estimated that 38 million persons do not have any insurance coverage, private or government, for health care costs. Nevertheless, even without information about this non-insured group, the picture is of widespread physical disability and chronic illness. Thus, however approximate, the available statistics suggest that chronic illness is a major and growing problem for large numbers of people in our society, limiting them in their daily activities.

Today, chronic illness is considered to be the number one health problem in our society by the United States Department of Health and Human Services. It creates a major public health issue in which the afflicted persons have to take major responsibility for managing their medical, social, and financial problems. Chronic illnesses, thus, tend to require fundamental readjustments on behalf of both the patient and of immediate caregivers, because these illnesses are of long duration with frequent exacerbations or recurrences; the victim may or may not die, but usually does not recover (e.g., in cases of diabetes, and arthritis). Indeed, these chronic illnesses last for a long time before the victims die. Usually, these illnesses cannot be cured, but the pain and suffering that they bring can be greatly reduced. To a certain extent, then, the emergence of chronic illnesses as today's big killers is, ironically, due to our medical success, increased longevity, and rising living standards.

FACTORS ASSOCIATED WITH PREVALENCE

Furthermore, chronic disorders are influenced by both environmental and behavioral factors. On the behavioral side, people choose to smoke or are unable to quit, thereby increasing their risk of heart problems and lung cancer; they eat too much, and/or knowingly or unknowingly eat the wrong kinds of foods, increasing their susceptibility to coronary disease and other problems. On the other hand, environmental factors influencing disease are even more complex and beyond most peoples' individual control. Consequently, medical factors alone are not enough to cure, much less prevent, the onset of today's predominant diseases.

Of course, changing and regulating certain health habits such as smoking, activity level, rest, and dietary intake may be easier to research and control; and they may well alter the course of certain conditions such as heart disease and chronic obstructive pulmonary disease. However, these health habits may not even be the primary causes of these and many other chronic health problems. Most chronically ill people do not necessarily display destructive health habits that are significantly different from those of non-chronically ill people. For instance, Syme (1975) has reported on studies in California and North Dakota that found rates of coronary heart disease twice as high among men who had experienced multiple job changes and geographic moves as among men with no such changes. The difference were attributable not to individual differences in diet, obesity, smoking and drinking habits, blood pressure, physical activity, age, or familial longevity, but to changes in the situation in which people lived, in other words, to environmental causes or socially induced stresses.

Moreover, there is danger in linking predisposing characteristics such as personality types and daily health care habits to the incidence and prevalence of chronic illness because it can easily lead to "victim blaming." Environmental causes responsible for so many chronic illnesses are beyond most peoples' individual control. As one of my respondents noted:

> And this humidity sometimes affects it, but I also find when I'm out in the country, 'cause I travel a lot in the mountains and that, that I can almost cut my medicine down to nothing because the air is so much. . . . In a city, I think it's just congestion and stuff. It really just closes and makes the lung problem worse. You know, . . . when I come back from my vacation . . . it's almost like having a culture shock, you know, 'cause my lungs, all of a sudden are shot back into needing the medication as where before I didn't need it.

I can really identify with what this respondent said, because for years I was blamed by those around me, including my doctor, for my asthmatic condition. I was told that the reason I was having problems was because either: "I didn't properly take care of myself. . . . I went out in the rain. . . . I was out in the evenings too much with my friends. . . . I didn't eat right. . . . I had a stressful job." My asthma disapeared in a miraculous manner, even though my stress level went up and none of my "bad habits" changed, when I emigrated to the United States from a totally different environment.

The study of the relationship between social factors and stress-related illnesses has advanced in the past two decades, but the precise nature of this relationship is not yet fully understood. It is clear from existing studies, however, that the experience of stress is a subjective response on the part of a person to certain social experiences. Undesirable life events cause the most stress, which, in turn, causes poorer health. McFarlane and colleagues (1983) found that events considered to be undesirable and not controllable by the respondents were consistently followed by an increase in reports of suffering, symptoms of illness, and physician visits. Having a chronic illness certainly falls in the category of undesirable life events. At the very least, even the cognition of having a chronic illness produces stress, which, in turn, causes poorer health, creating a vicious cycle.

The relationship between stress and life events as a precipitating or contributing factor in chronic illnesses is a highly complex phenomenon and not easily amenable to simple cause-and-effect explanations. Most chronic illnesses, in fact, begin without the afflicted person's awareness of significant physiologic changes.

As Dimond and Jones (1983, p. 636) note, "Neither the incidence nor the prevalence of chronic conditions is a sufficient indication of the magnitude of the problem. The real measure is the extent to which individuals with chronic illness and their families are functioning in ways that are acceptable to them." Indeed, a chronic illness can make a person's life miserable and profoundly affect the lives of those around them.

In sum, the prevalence of chronic illness has risen as the environments we live in have become more polluted and complex, and as the population has aged and acute disease has come under greater control. Because of biomedical and technologic advances, more people are being kept alive, if not cured, from previously fatal conditions. Thus, the good news is that these killer illnesses are now much less likely to kill, at least initially; the bad news is that medical success has brought new meaning to the chronicity of these conditions.

ECONOMIC BURDEN OF CHRONIC ILLNESS

In an interview to the media on September 6, 1990, Dr. Louis Sullivan, health and human services secretary, noted that the United States spent $600 billion on health care in 1989, and he said that if the same pattern is followed, the bill would be $1.5 trillion by the year 2000. Health care is the largest service industry in the United States, and Americans spend over $1,000 billion annually on health—more than 14 percent of their personal income (Taylor 1995).

According to National Center for Health Statistics (1996), in 1980, an average of $1,063 per person was spent on health care in the United States; by 1994 this figure had risen to $3,510 —the highest in the world. The next highest, Switzerland (based upon 1993 figures), spent $2,283 per person on health compared to $3,221 for the United States. Also in 1980, Americans spent a total of $250.1 billion on health needs, as compared to 1994 expenditures of $949.4 billion. Hospital costs alone in 1994 were $338.5 billion, and the total amount of expenditures for physician services in the same year was $189.4 billion.

The share of gross national product spent on health care in our country is also higher than in other industrial countries, soaring from under 5 percent in the early 1950s to over 13 percent in 1992. Furthermore, some 8.9 percent of the gross domestic products (GDP) was spent on health in 1980, increasing to 13.7 percent in 1994. To emphasize the increase and magnitude of the cost of health care in American society, we can examine the U.S. consumer price index. According to that measure, between 1984 and 1995 the cost of medical care increased by 140.5 percent, more than any other major category of personal expense.

Indeed, the United States medical system remains, by far, the most expensive in the world, yet Americans are not the healthiest people in the world. For instance, 20 countries have lower infant mortality rates, and 21 have longer life expectancies (Population Reference Bureau 1991). However, as already mentioned, mortality statistics do not reflect the amount of morbidity present in a society. Conditions such as rheumatoid arthritis and osteoarthritis have little impact on mortality rates but a major impact on the functioning and well-being of the population, particularly the elderly population. Morbidity rates, a better indicator of the health status of a population, also happen to be very high in American society, as discussed in the previous section.

Specifically, the burden of chronic illness upon society's resources is reported as 57 percent of the national expenditure for health care, 59 percent of hospital days, and 60 percent of all economic costs, direct and indirect (U.S. DHEW 1979). In fact, medical costs keep spiraling upward at the rate of about 10 percent a year, well above the 5 percent rate of inflation.

There are many factors contributing to this situation. One is the development of new and more expensive technology requiring highly trained workers to operate the new equipment and perform the new procedures. It is ironic that, contrary to the economic principle of supply and demand, the growing number of doctors in the United States boosts health care costs instead of lowering these costs. A possible explanation might be that young doctors, eager to attract patients, are quick to offer the new high-tech treatments, which can only be performed in hospitals, adding to the cost. Older doctors must then do the same to stay competitive, so the nation's health care bill rises ever higher. In fact, an important feature that distinguishes our health care system from those of other industrial societies is the ability of American physicians to set their own fees. In most other countries the initiation of third-party payment was accompanied by cost controls that limited the fees that could be charged and reviewed the necessity of proposed medical procedures. In our country, this did not happen until the 1980s, and still has occurred to a lesser extent than in other countries. Analyzing American medicine from a conflict and historical perspective, sociologist Paul Starr (1982) has attributed this difference to the great political power of doctors and hospitals in the United States.

Another reason for spiraling costs is the rise of defensive medicine, which is the ordering of medical tests and procedures by doctors to head off malpractice suits. The American Medical Association estimates that defensive medicine costs between $12 billion and $14 billion a year (Marshall 1990). A related reason is the cost of malpractice insurance, which rose enormously in recent decades, as more and more people sued physicians for treatment that went wrong. In 1990, American doctors paid $4.5 billion in malpractice premiums. This extra cost is paid by all insured doctors—good, bad, or medio-cre—and it is inevitably passed on to patients.

A major reason for increasing costs is the aging (and therefore more chronically ill) population. Older people, in general, use more medical services than younger ones. Between 1940 and 1990, the proportion of the population that is elderly nearly doubled, from about 7 to 12 percent. This trend will continue as the baby-boom generation ages. By year 2030 an estimated 25 percent of our population will be elderly, a fact that has ominous implications for the total cost of health care.

Last but not least, another reason for the increase in health care costs is that American health care is essentially a system of interven-tion rather than prevention; the system is oriented toward treating and curing disease rather than preventing it. As a result the majority of Americans do not usually come into contact with the health care system unless they become ill. When this happens, the health care providers they come in contact with are often highly trained specialists who use the most advanced technology to provide treatment—if the patient can afford it. Thus, the system can accurately be described as more of a medical care system rather than a true health care system.

Furthermore, the American system of medical care has at least two tiers. One is for the well-off and well-insured: the upper classes, the elderly through Medicare, the middle class with "good" jobs at large companies, and government employees. Military personnel, their families, and veterans are taken care of by separate government-sponsored and government-controlled health care systems. A second tier is for the poor who are eligible for government-funded Medicaid. And there is no system at all for approximately 38 million American citizens with no insurance and too little income to afford a serious illness, particularly long-term chronic illness. Indeed, American health care suffers from "the inverse coverage law": the more people need insurance coverage, the less likely they are to get it (Light 1990).

Since access to the health care system is highly unequal, being based on the ability to pay, many of the uninsured have to forgo preventive health care in the form of routine checkups and screening. As a result, their health problems go undetected until they are well advanced and more expensive to treat. Thus, when the uninsured get seriously ill for a long period of time, they are often forced to go begging for treatment, usually in hospital emergency rooms, hoping that doctors and public hospitals will not turn them away or give them inadequate treatment.

Furthermore, these people not only may not get the care they need, but also place a financial burden on taxpayers, hospitals, and other patients. In 1988, unpaid hospital bills alone amounted to over $8 billion (Consumer Reports 1990). Hospitals and doctors who care for the uninsured typically raise the fees they charge insured patients and those with Medicare or Medicaid, in an effort to compensate for their losses.

Medicare and Medicaid are the largest payers of medical bills, $79.9 billion in the fiscal year 1987. A report from the Health Care Financing Administration (Nov. 18, 1988) concluded by stating: "It is imperative that we identify the most effective means of providing health care to avoid unnecessary and duplicate procedures." In 1997, we were still attempting to do that, and we are still debating.

The foregoing discussion about the high costs of health care has great relevance to chronically ill people because, although all people are possible targets of chronic illness and the largest number of victims is under 65 years of age, older persons are more likely to be disabled by chronic conditions, in many cases suffering from more than one, and have less resources to deal with them.   Since the proportion of older persons in the population of the United States is growing, chronic illnesses will become an ever increasing problem, contributing greatly to the economic impoverishment of the individual people involved, as well as becoming an even greater drain on societal resources. For example, in 1984, Medicare alone paid out $15 billion for the treatment of chronically ill Americans in the last six months of their lives; that is more than the entire gross national product of many developing countries. Yet it is a modest amount considering the latest increases in health care expenditures.

Part of the problem is that doctors in the United States, more than elsewhere in the world, try aggressively to keep hospitalized terminally ill patients and even brain-dead patients alive on machines, often against their wishes and those of their families, while at the same time neglecting the needs of the less seriously ill, home-based chronically ill persons. For instance, a respondent who quit nursing after twelve years, partially because of her illness explained:

> And it's just not worth it anymore! Not, emotionally, not for me, it's not! And I don't enjoy it. I enjoy taking care of the elderly people and that, but not to the point we're gonna have to go out of our way to try and push somebody who's 89 years old and just does not want to be pushed anymore. I mean, and there's a time in everybody's life when you die and that's it. And a lot of hospitals and a lot of doctors, due to the fact that they want the money, seem to forget this. And I can't deal with it!

At the present time, despite the enormous amounts paid by Medicare and Medicaid, those persons in our society with chronic health problems are experiencing many hardships due to reduced funding of necessary programs in an age of economic and regulatory pressures.

Medicare and Medicaid remain substantially medicalized, in the sense that provided care is primarily either directly medical, under medical supervision, or certified by physicians. Thus, these financial controls continue to reinforce care that is offered in an institutional context, making the development of noninstitutional or home-based health care provisions virtually impossible. The resulting effect is inconsistent with the needs of chronically ill persons, regardless of their social and economic positions. These needs are only partially medical, but mostly social, psychological, and financial.

In the United States, we spend much time, many resources, and great effort on determining eligibility for publicly supported services. To be entitled to Medicaid, the principal source of nationally supported long-term care, chronically ill persons have to produce documentation of financial impoverishment. It is ironic that a person needing long-term care who is not initially entitled by poverty or age to receive Medicaid and/or Medicare support may, as a result of personal payment for that care, become impoverished enough to be eligible for Medicaid or Medicare, as the following example illustrates.

He was a nice doctor! I had no complaints! Only, he charged me too much, that's the only problem! Charged me $6,500. . . . They charge $1,500 a month for dialysis, but now I have Medicare. I don't have to pay. Medicare pays 80 percent and Public Health Department pays the other 20 percent. But when I first went to the hospital, I didn't have Medicare because I still wasn't of age. I was 60 years old. I still, you know, you have to be about 65. So I didn't have Medicare. I didn't have hospitalization. I ended up owing the hospital $35,000, and their different doctors did different operations. . . . And, so I owe $15,000 to the doctors. . . . I paid this; between the hospital and the doctors, I paid $5,000. So, I still owe — well it was $35 [thousand] hospital, $15 [thousand] doctors and then technicians, like neurology, radiology, and X-rays, that was another $5,000. . . . I have to pay. I have to pay what happened at that time. Now, they pay! So I paid $5,000, and I had some money in the bank, but I didn't know how I was going to pay the rent, though. And they want the money. They said they'll take me to court and . . . they send me threatening letters. . . . Well, I try to give every month a little bit at a time, like $50, $100. . . . But, I only get $250 a month disability, and, well, I get also $250 policeman part. My husband was a policeman. And I do get Social Security, but only $34 a month. So that's not much. The rent is over $300 over here, and then I have to pay for cab fare. Even if I get rides it costs me still $100 a month for cab fare. Then, $100 for food. . . . I mean, it's terrible to be sick and still have this hanging over you that's — You have to pay all that money or they are going to make trouble for you. So it's not easy!

The $100 a month cab fare this 62-year-old respondent is talking about is for going to the dialysis center three times a week, when her children are unable to take her there because of their conflicting work schedules. Of course, there are some bus services available for disabled people, but these services are limited and not very reliable for persons who have to be on time for their allotted period on a dialysis machine or lose their turn. Thus as she says, "It's not easy!"

Even people living in rural communities, with more "community or neighborly help" available to them, seem to have a hard time dealing with the financial burdens of chronic illness. I went out of my way to find and interview a chronically ill person living in a nonurban environment, and found a woman, age 65, who lives alone in a rural Illinois town. She has diabetes, heart disease, and crippling arthritis, in addition to poor circulation and sinus problems. She recalled that her problems began about 15 or 20 years ago when she finally sought a doctor and was diagnosed as a "borderline diabetic" and put on medication. She tried very hard to keep her job as a machine operator at a local plant, but finally had to quit after two years because her poor health caused her to miss too many days of work. Her problems multiplied when, eight years later, she suffered a severe heart attack that placed her in the hospital for 27 days, 10 of which were in intensive care.

At the time of the interview, this woman was taking many different medications for her heart, arthritis, and diabetes problems. She was seeing two doctors, one a surgeon and general internist, the other a cardiologist whom she saw as needed, or every three months for checkups. She also had to see what she called a "bone specialist" once or twice a year, and if she required any other special treatment, she was sent to a specialist in a city 40 miles away. It took me by surprise that despite her massive health problems, what seemed to bother this respondent most were her financial burdens caused by her ill health, her dependence on other people because of her financial situation, and the fact that she could not do many of the things she previously enjoyed, such as fishing. She stated that she had worked most of her life and at the present time had to try to survive on the very minimal Social Security Disability benefits she receives (totaling only $453 a month). She also has a "red, white, and blue card," which covers 80 percent of her hospital and doctor bills, but does not cover the cost of her prescriptions, which average about $190 to $200 a month. Because she receives a few dollars too many from Social Security Disability, she is not eligible for a year-round welfare medical card that covers all medications. Instead, she had a "spend-down" of $414, and only after she reached this could she receive the "medical card." She could use this only for four or five months, and then it was taken away again until she reached the "spend-down" once more. During those months when she had to pay for prescriptions on her own, she could not afford to pay her gas, electric, food, and telephone bills. Thus, her medicine was bought on credit from the local druggist who "ups the price of every item by a dollar or a dollar-and-a-half." She noted that when she purchased it on the medical card, there were limits to how much the druggist could charge, but not when she was paying out of her pocket. She nevertheless could not switch to another store because this was the only place she could get credit. Most of the time, she had to pay her utility bills in partial payments and was also limited in her choice of grocery stores. To buy food, only one store allowed her to pay with a postdated check after her monthly $10 in food stamps ran out.

She noted that her doctors were "nice and tolerant" because they knew her personally, were aware of her financial situation, and knew that she would pay whatever she could when her checks came in each month. It was her friends and neighbors, though, who gave her the most help: bringing her the mail from the box a half-mile down the road, taking turns to call her on the phone each day, bringing her home-cooked meals periodically, and taking her to the doctor whenever she needed to go. She has also had some help from two separate Homecare programs that send a nurse every two weeks to take blood samples to regulate her insulin intake.

This respondent has learned that she must accept the cumulative effects of her illnesses and depend on other people if she is to survive; she expressed feelings of gratitude for those who help her out. She noted that she could not have survived this long if it was not for all the help she has received, yet it is not the biological ailments that seem to harm her the most. The financial problems as well as the stressful psychological burdens make the physical effects of her chronic illnesses all the worse. In fact, the respondent reported that when she "gives in, usually at the end of each month," all of her health problems become aggravated; she tries consciously to avoid thinking about all the bills, since these thoughts produce stress that in turn causes her more health problems. But the bills and reminders keep coming. As a respondent quoted earlier said, "It's not easy!"

Many respondents talked about financial difficulties and their fears about being "a burden" to their families and friends. For example, discussing the economic burden placed on chronically ill persons and their families by an ongoing illness condition, a condition that affects and worries everybody regardless of their socioeconomic status, one of my more affluent respondents had an interesting way of expressing his financial concerns: "I want to point out to you, there's a great deal of difference between dead and economic dead! When you're dead, you're dead! All the expenses stop and the insurance comes in. When you suffer economic dead, all the expenses go on or increase, you see!"

When asked about her main concerns in dealing with a chronic illness, a health care professional, a nurse with access to all sorts of resources, said:

And the other thing, like I said, [that] is very hard to deal with is the expense. Medication is so expensive. . . . I have hospitalization at—Since they cut down benefits and that, it doesn't cover my medicine that I buy every month now, and that can run anywhere from forty to fifty dollars a month. A month! My mother's cost a hundred and thirty five dollars a month. . . . So, that all comes out of my pocket and I find that financially—that's money I could be using to do other things with, and it bothers me that drugs cost so much. Even if it's generic, . . . it just costs an arm and a leg to keep your supply of drugs.

The point of all this is that all respondents I interviewed talked at length about the immense pressure they are under because of the continuous debts created by their chronic health problems. Nobody is arguing that professional services should be without costs or meet all needs. They cannot and, in any case, neither chronically ill persons nor their families expect the professionals to have all the answers or solutions, particularly to needs in the social and psychological domains; nor do they expect these professionals to work for no fees. Rather, the point is to identify ways of furthering the self-care expertise of chronically ill people and their families, by enhancing their adaptive skills and providing needed information and resources directly to them instead of keeping them so dependent on health care professionals. Chronically ill people, just like everybody else, need to feel that they have some control over their lives, including their illness and its consequences. Thus, as Dimond and Jones (1983, p. 650) state, "chronic illness is a major health problem. The cost in terms of healthcare dollars and loss of employment is staggering; but the cost to individual lives in terms of pain, distress, despair, and disruption of families is overwhelming."

Chronic illnesses are also expensive to treat, particularly when those illnesses persist for years, even decades. The effects that chronic illnesses involving dysfunction have on medical costs may well be underestimated in current policy analyses of health care costs and cost-effectiveness (Kaplan, Coons, & Anderson 1992).

Part I

Characteristics and Consequences of Chronic Illness

> When you find out that you are ill, your priorities are shattered. One moment you are in a boat, and the next moment you are in the water.
>
> —Susan Sontag

According to Maddox and Glass (1989), chronic illnesses are characterized by low "specificity," meaning the absence of definitive etiology, natural course, and distinct interventions. They are also often categorized as having an "ambiguous identity," that is, unlike acute illnesses, the symptoms of chronic conditions may be nonspecific, intermittent, and thus difficult to identify. A respondent in my study said:

> I really hadn't had any physical problems. The only thing that I can think of is that when I was in college I had problems with hamstring muscle pulls, and I had to go to the doctor there to get—so I didn't have to go to a PE class. . . . I was playing intramural football and . . . I mentioned to the doctor that if I sat too long—that if I'm driving down to school and if I sat too long—that I would have to get out of the car because my legs would be real stiff and sore; they would really throb and hurt.

And he just said something about, well, maybe a blood disorder
of some type and I'd have to see my regular GP, a regular doctor
at home about it, after that. I had been fairly healthy up to then.
Matter of fact, I think I had been in the hospital once in my life
after I was born, and that's when I was very young and they
thought — it was nothing major — it was nothing special! No
suggestion of MS! . . . The doctor was kind of worried because
mine went so progressively fast, from being perfectly — I thought
perfectly — healthy and then a month later to have to use crutches
to even get around, period! And even then I couldn't stay up too
long on crutches; my legs were very, very weak.

Most chronic illnesses seem to begin without the afflicted person's
awareness of significant physiologic changes:

I, after 18 years old, from 18 up until two years ago, never went
to the doctor. I was just in perfect health! I was used to doing
everything, so when that happened [she had a hysterectomy], I
would go to work and drag myself home and go to sleep. So
then, after I got out of the hospital, I was great until one morning
in July I woke up and Oh God! I couldn't even explain it. Just
every part of my body hurt so bad, and I went to get up and I
thought I had a stroke. I screamed for J. to come help me 'cause
I couldn't get out of bed and the arthritis just didn't dawn on me.
I just thought that either they botched up my operation somehow
or I had a stroke, and I couldn't figure it out.

An individual may be conscious of a condition (e.g., rheumatoid
arthritis) but dismiss it as "normal wear and tear" of the aging
process, or be completely unaware of any disorder (e.g., diabetes or
hypertension). In many cases, the diagnosis of a chronic illness takes
a long time, sometimes years.
    As an extreme example, one respondent who suffers from severe
multiple sclerosis thought that most of the unusual symptoms, such as
the off-and-on blindness she initially experienced, were due to her
pregnancy at the time. She was reinforced in that belief when her
doctors could not come up with other possible explanations for it and
also thought that her difficulties were related to her pregnancy. She
was misdiagnosed for a few years, going through another pregnancy
with very serious symptoms before the health care experts realized that

she had been suffering for years from multiple sclerosis without receiving any medical treatment for it.

Other respondents related similar, if less serious, experiences. Some of them said that they were accused of laziness or drunkenness when in actuality they were displaying symptoms of serious chronic illnesses. For instance, a younger respondent related how difficult it was for her to convince first her parents and then her doctor that she was seriously suffering from asthma:

> I pretty much figured before them that I had asthma, but you know, I was only like 12, 13. And grown-ups were telling me: no, you don't have it! You don't have asthma. So, I knew that I had asthma. . . . I don't know if I knew it was asthma, but I just knew that I had trouble breathing and it wasn't from an allergy. . . . My brother and I both had cases where, you know, we used to run around a lot and play a lot, and after that we had trouble breathing and we couldn't catch our breath. . . . I guess maybe, we were 10? 9? . . . And for a long time, my dad just thought, you know, it was, "Oh! it's nothing! Maybe you're just playing too hard or whatever." And, then after that, you know, he finally realized that I had a problem. . . . Um, well, my dad first realized it was really a problem when I was about 15, 12 or 15. . . . When I finally found out? Well, I think I was kinda relieved more than anything else. I thought, Good, they finally thought it was what I thought it was, so they gave me the right medicine for it and it helped me out a lot. I felt kinda relived when I found out that the doctors finally agreed with what I was saying it was.

Even if people are aware of their symptoms, sometimes they are not believed by others. At first, it was hard for me to believe that most of my respondents indicated that they had no prior warnings or symptoms of their illness before they were diagnosed. That surprised me and consequently prompted me to seek out and interview health-care professionals who also happen to suffer from some chronic illness, thinking that these people, trained in the art of diagnosis, might be more aware of their bodily states. Yet even these respondents, who were doctors and nurses, indicated that they had no prior awareness of their illness before they were, as one put it, "hit with it." Does a chronic illness really hit suddenly, or are people denying the warnings or symptoms until they can no longer do so and have to get medical help? Only one respondent openly admitted her denial:

> I should have been to the hospital when I first discovered that lump . . . because I was basically scared that it was cancer, and I didn't want to hear it! What scared me the most? Finding out if it really was cancer, basically, because all my family had died so far with cancer and I just knew eventually it was going to hit home, hit me! And, I didn't want to hear, I did not want to hear that word CANCER! I was playing games with myself.

In fact, denial is a defense mechanism by which people avoid the implications of a serious illness. They pretend that their illness is acute, a temporary condition, and ignore medical information that contradicts it. In other words, people want to believe that their lives will go on exactly as before, even though they now have a permanent impairment. Denial is a common reaction to chronic illness that has been observed among heart patients (Krantz & Deckel 1983), stroke patients (Diller 1976), and cancer patients (Katz, Weiner, Gallagher, & Hellman 1970; Levine & Zigler 1975; Meyerowitz 1983).

Another possible explanation for not recognizing an illness, as noted by Rodin (1978, p. 532), is that people often get imprecise and vague feedback from their physical states, especially when everything is working smoothly: "Even when something feels wrong, the discomfort may be hard to identify. Not only are perceived symptoms ambiguous, but they are typically unfamiliar. When symptoms are difficult to evaluate objectively, they lead to even more speculative inferences than occur normally, which may make for possibly erroneous perceptions."

Charmaz (1991, p. 17) also notes that having a chronic illness is ambiguous in many ways, that "people hold sketchy and simplistic conceptions of their illness," and that doctors also feed into these misconceptions. Thus many times what looks like denial may simply be an initial response by a patient who lacks information and understanding about his or her diagnosis. In fact, Charmaz perceptively points out that "professionals sometimes make hasty judgments of denial during fleeting encounters with bewildered, shocked, or fearful patients, who cannot communicate, or perhaps even articulate, their concerns at the time" (p. 17).

When symptoms are ambiguous, they also lead to speculative inferences about the character of the sufferers by their significant others. For example, a couple of respondents mentioned that they were actually relieved when they were finally diagnosed, even with a serious illness, because at least it stopped people around them from accusing them, in one case, of being a "secret drinker," and in another case, of being a "hypochondriac."

Recognition of physical symptoms is difficult to evaluate objectively and, in fact, varies from culture to culture. Payer (1988), a medical journalist who has written on "cultural biases in medicine," notes that people in different cultures attribute their illnesses to different causes. For instance, the French attribute most of their problems to dysfunction of the liver, the Germans to the heart. She further notes that:

> the same clinical signs may even receive different diagnoses. Often, all one must do to acquire a disease is to enter a country where that disease is recognized—leaving the country will either cure the malady or turn it into something else. . . . World travelers who have had to see a doctor in a foreign country have usually discovered that medicine is not quite the international science that the medical profession would like us to believe. Not only do ways of delivering medical care differ from country to country, so does the medicine that is delivered. The differences are so great that one country's treatment of choice may be considered malpractice across the border. . . . One World Health Organization study found that doctors from different countries diagnosed different causes of death even when shown identical information from the same death certificates. (Payer 1988, pp. 24–25)

Culturally, situations that focus attention on the body may also lead to an increased awareness of physical problems (Pennebaker 1982). For example, national publicity given to breast cancer in public figures such as First Ladies Betty Ford and Nancy Reagan may make individual women more likely to perform self-examinations and/or seek medical attention.

Recognition of physical symptoms may also vary from individual to individual within a given culture. According to Scheier, Carver, and Gibbons (1979), people who score high on a dimension of "private self-consciousness" are more likely to detect physical symptoms.

"Self-consciousness" is defined as a disposition to focus attention inward on the self and can be further analyzed in terms of its public and private aspects. "Private self-consciousness" involves a focus on personal aspects of the self, such as bodily sensations, beliefs, moods, and feelings. People who score high on measures of this dimension are more aware of their internal feelings and are quicker to make self-descriptive statements (Carver 1979; Mueller 1982). Such people also tend to be aware of changes in their bodily states, and may tend to be healthier than others because they can recognize stresses to their bodies and take action before the stress is physically damaging (Mullen & Suls 1982).

Awareness of one's symptoms, however, does not always lead to an immediate search for medical attention. Often the factors to which an individual attributes symptoms hinder the quest for medical expertise (Rodin 1978; Taylor 1982). Frequent stomach pains may be self-diagnosed as a minor case of tension or nerves rather than a severe ulcer. In fact, judgments of the severity of a medical problem are biased when the illness is one's own. These judgments are also influenced by beliefs about the prevalence of the illness in question.

> Blood pressure considered treatably high in the United States might be considered normal in England; and the low blood pressure treated with eighty-five drugs as well as hydrotherapy and spa treatments in Germany would entitle its sufferer to lower life insurance rates in the United States. The differences are most marked for minor complaints but not at all limited to them. "Plenty of people," wrote Dr. M. N. G. Dukes in *British Medical Journal,* "are still dying of diseases which other people do not believe in." (Payer 1988, p. 25)

Hence both of these factors, one concerning "personal relevance" and the other about the "prevalence of the illness" in society, influence the judgment people make of the severity of the condition, and that, in turn, determines whether they will seek medical attention. For example, AIDS was not perceived to be a threat to health in general when it was initially prevalent only in a small segment of the population, particularly a population that most people did not consider relevant to themselves. In other words, people who believe relatively few people have the condition consider it a less serious threat to health than people who think many people have that same condition.

Furthermore, if these same people believe that they themselves have the condition, they consider it, for whatever reason, to be significantly less serious. A 42-year-old respondent recalled his first reactions upon being told about his diagnosis:

> This is going to sound strange. I was relieved, only because I was afraid it was something more drastic. I was somewhat familiar with it—not as much as I should have been—only because I had two neighbors I know that had it [multiple sclerosis]. So, it wasn't so disastrous on the sense that the two neighbors I know that had it—as far as I know—well, one had died recently now, but she died of some other ailment. I knew it was not necessarily life threatening. The idea of what it could have been! The doctor was talking about surgery—I was more afraid of other things. . . . Well, a tumor. It could have been a tumor in the brain; it could have been a tumor in the spine. And so knowing that it was something that I could possibly live with, I was somewhat relieved I wasn't too pleased, in the sense that I wished that I had nothing at all.

Although this respondent had two neighbors who suffered from multiple sclerosis, he still considered the illness relatively uncommon and apparently not very serious; he went searching for medical attention because he thought that he had what he considered to be a "real" problem, such as a tumor in the brain or spine, an even more uncommon occurrence but with more personal relevance to himself. He elaborated that he had a cousin that "has since died, because they can't—the brain tumors—they don't get it all; . . . they try to operate and they could not get it all. He lived a few years, but then it just took over."

Equally important, then, people interpret symptoms according to their knowledge, perceptions, and past experiences with health matters. They are also quite defensive about their own health. In many cases this defensiveness about their own health, like the behavior of the person who ignores persistent stomach problems or dismisses a potential skin cancer as a bad case of sunburn, causes serious delays in the search for treatment, often leading to more serious health problems. As Charmaz (1991, p.18) points out, "The more esoteric the illness, the more likely the person initially lacks information and understanding about it."

The ambigious identity of chronic illness aside, the most frequently mentioned problems in living with chronic illness, according to my data, seem to center around the experiences of "uncertainty" and "stigma," and the most devastating consequence appears to be "social isolation." In various ways, all my respondents talked about these aspects of chronic illness more than anything else, because these aspects impact the most on their quality of life. Quality of life is a multidimensional construct, involving not only physical functioning, stamina, absence of pain, control of symptoms, and self-care ability, but also coping ability, adjustment to illness, role functioning, life satisfaction, and usefulness to others (Jalowiec 1990). As can be seen, quality of life deals with two separate but related sets of needs: (1) the need to avoid, diminish, and/or adjust to distressing life experiences, and (2) the need to develop and sustain life satisfaction by increasing competence and mastery over one's environment (Holmes 1989).

In recent years the assessment of quality of life has shifted mainly from reliance on objective indicators of physical functioning to a consideration of psychological, social, and economic factors. For example, Pearlman and Uhlmann (1988), in their study of the perceptions of elderly patients with the five most common chronic illnesses, found that quality of life was largely based on these patients' perception of their health, interpersonal relationships, and finances. It is interesting to note that these chronically ill people saw themselves in more optimistic terms and as more functionally advantaged than did their doctors, who saw them more in terms of their diseases.

In fact, there is increasing recognition among health care specialists that quality of life, although a subjective experience that can best be rated by chronically ill persons themselves, is an important health outcome with major implications for compliance with medical treatments. For some illnesses, such as arthritis, quality of life is the important health outcome.

In fact, near the completion of the interview, when I asked my respondents, "Overall, how has having [name of the illness] affected your life?" They all talked about the social aspects rather than their medical problems. For example, one respondent answered:

How has it affected my life? It took me away from . . . what I love doing, for which I was very highly compensated. It has limited to an extent what I can do physically. It has created an infinite amount of boredom! But to be honest, I'm sincere when I say, what have I got to complain about? What have I got to complain about? . . . I'm going from a top level executive with a six-figure income, I go from that overnight, now overnight, the surgery was February . . . at the end of April . . . and when they said don't ever go back to your office, and overnight I went from indispensable to nothing!

A homemaker and mother of four expressed the same sentiments:

I just felt, what was I gonna do, I had no occupation. My whole life was my children and my home. I already was not able to do it full caliber, but I would manage. Then, to have this thrown at me! I was like: what is there left for me to do? Now, I'm not able to do anything! . . . Something else to do beside watch the dumb TV. I hate TV! I turn it on, I don't know why, But uh, I just get to a point where I'm going to scream! I can't stand another commercial!

The presence of a chronic illness significantly alters a person's everyday behavior and gives rise to much disability, loss of earning capacity, need for constant medical care, and, perhaps even more important, a decrease in the quality and fullness of life. As one of my less incapacitated respondents, who is able to live a reasonably "normal" life, nevertheless wistfully noted:

Probably the thing that's the least fine is just accepting the fact that I can't, you know, I can't go bike riding with R. up the hills or anything without having the cardiac problem set in. My husband was in an aerobics class at work. After work, R. went up there a couple of times with him. I would take her up there. She could exercise . . . and I found myself semijealous and a little bit sad that I knew I couldn't do that with them.

The determinants of quality of life are independent of disease categories and age. These respondents talked about their medical problems, financial problems, and frustrations with health care professionals, particularly about the fact that they were not getting much help from these professionals. As one of my respondents, after seeing many specialists for her condition, stated, "They don't tell you

right out, but you get the point. . . . They can't do anything for you."
Sometimes they do "tell you right out," as another one of my respondents recalled:

> I was getting, I would say what you would call attacks which
> lasted about a week to ten days. . . . Then I started with a—well,
> I had the orthopedic man, then I went to a man who just handled
> arthritis, to double check, because this orthopedic surgeon said I
> had arthritis. Well, I figured why not go to somebody who all
> they do is just arthritis and maybe he's got something that'll help
> me. I went there, and he said there's nothing that can be done! It's
> definitely arthritis, and you have to live with it!

Almost everybody is told, one way or another, "to learn to live
with it," since there is no cure for these chronic conditions, at our
present state of knowledge. People accept that definition; what they
are mostly frustrated about is the fact that they are not getting much
help from health care professionals in how to do it. There seems to
be a gap between peoples' expectations about the kinds of help they
feel they should be getting from these professionals and what they are
getting in reality, which these chronically ill people feel is not much.
Part of the reason is that, in many cases, professionals themselves do
not have all the answers. The ill are constantly exposed to
contradictory research findings, and the contradictions are compounded
by the way medical science itself is constantly changing.

In fact, a couple of my chronically ill respondents who also happen
to be nurses indicated that doctors are not always up on the latest
medical findings, and therefore many patients do not get adequate
care. These nurses became particularly aware of this fact when they
cared for patients who had the same illness they have. As one of them
stated:

> I find it very hard to take care of a pulmonary case only because
> I know what can happen. . . . And it's very difficult for me, when
> I'm yelling at a doctor: I think you need to put vitamins in his
> I.V. You know, they keep massive doses of steroids and . . . you
> better start giving him vitamins so it can absorb . . . and espe-
> cially with a lot of young doctors and that, they think they know
> it all and they get out of med school and they don't want to listen
> to you! I've gotten myself in trouble several times with doctors

and that because I've stood my ground, you know, but it's always turned out I've been right! . . . My obsession for vitamins, but I know from my own case, that this was what was going to help. So, I went ahead and got a, what we call a latch, from the library on the disease and on the new studies that have been done, and I brought it down, and he's [the doctor is] standing there and I showed it to him. . . . And the doctor started giving me all kinds of hassle.

Another respondent, who had been a general practitioner for over twenty years before he was diagnosed with kidney failure, stated that he never realized before how patients felt about not being informed, and how they were treated "as morons . . . yes, even me!" by health care professionals. Thus, besides a decrease in quality of life, one of the consequences of chronic illness seems to be the frustration chronically ill people feel in their interactions with health care professionals.

Chronic illness does affect an afflicted person's body image, sexual functioning, psychological well-being, social identity, and occupational role. A very active and dynamic man, who described himself as a "type A personality," forced to retire at the height of his career because of a chronic heart condition, noted:

I'd love to walk the golf course! Riding a golf course is just– I haven't been able to walk a golf course in years. I'd like very much to be able to go back to work, but I know I can't 'cause of my health. But, I don't have to go back to work, so I really don't think about it in any regressive sense, because there's no financial requirement. . . . I miss people! Through my business, I directly or indirectly had a partial effect on the lives of over 300,000 people, through 125 corporations. . . . I was an employee benefit consultant. I designed pension, profit sharing plans, so forth and etcetera, for industry. And I very much miss that! No, I don't miss getting on a train and going downtown or driving down.

On the other hand, a respondent with a severe heart condition and other related complications who also has no "financial requirements" to work and could in fact voluntarily retire very comfortably because his son is the CEO of the corporation, nevertheless shows up at work almost every day, involving himself with a lot of high level corporate matters. This respondent, age 62, discussed many reasons why he persists in working despite his physical problems. To paraphrase him, his social identity and psychological well-being depend on it.

At the minimum, for many persons, the diagnosis of a chronic illness forces an awareness of a permanent defect, however slight, and the need to learn how to live with something less than the accustomed level of functioning that was previously taken for granted. One respondent summarized the feelings expressed by many people: "I'm adjusting to it, but at first, you feel like your life is all over."

Indeed, the diagnosis of a chronic illness often comes as a tremendous shock to a person. Within a few hours, there is a recognition that many plans may have to change and the life course adjusted. In fact, I hypothesized that since becoming ill, particularly with a long-term, chronic illness, inevitably results in drastic changes in an individual's physical and social functioning and role behavior, it would almost force that individual to examine the assumptions about the self and others previously taken-for-granted. In other words, I thought that getting chronically ill would lead to concentrated efforts of self perception.

The data I collected support my notion that many people learn a great deal about themselves, or at least maintain that they do so, when they become seriously ill and confront their own mortality. At the very least, for most of them, becoming chronically ill leads to a change of priorities. Many of these chronically ill people interviewed said that they turned to religion for answers. For instance, the "Why me?" question was raised by many respondents before I even had a chance to ask them. I was particularly fascinated by peoples' perception of God. It was as though they were talking about a "celestial vending machine" with so much input versus so much expected output: "I'm a good person, and I always went to church, so why did this happen to me?" and "I don't understand — why me? I don't really deserve this from God!" were the kinds of reactions expressed by most people interviewed.

However, realizing that maybe God operates rather like a "celestial slot machine," that bad things do indeed happen randomly to good people, seems greatly to unsettle and disturb most of these chronically ill people. Some of them even display anger: "Why me? Why me? I can't honestly — you know, that's this! That's shaking your fist! I

can't honestly answer . . . that! Well, I'm shaking my fist to God."
Another respondent said:

> After you get over feeling sorry for yourself—'cause that's a first
> reaction—then I'd get angry, and I think after the anger passes,
> Angry at what? At the world! At God! Why me? You know,
> why does this have to happen? What did I do that I should have
> to suffer so much? I felt real sorry for myself because I said, look,
> God, I went through— My husband had a bleeding ulcer and
> almost died—I went throught that. My father died when I was—
> You know, what else do you want?

In general, most people seem rather philosophical and conciliatory,
yet they all seem to search for answers, for some hidden meaning.
Indeed, the oldest idea of what causes illness is that it is a punishment.
As Sontag (1989, p. 2) notes, the belief that "illness reveals, and is a
punishment for, moral laxity or turpitude" creates a metaphor that
stands in the way of treatment and cure.

As the prominent social psychologist Kelley (1973, p. 108) noted,
"Causal attributions play an important role in providing the impetus to
action and decision among alternative courses of action." Indeed, the
attribution process itself has consequences for the ill person, because
the person may put off seeking proper medical attention while
engaging in a search for explanation and causation. As one of my
respondents recalled: "I had back problems, off and on, always.
Yeah, I thought it was flaring up. I couldn't walk! I couldn't do
anything! I was flat on my back for two weeks before we finally gave
in to the fact that they were going to have to do something."

The most important question about attributions for chronically ill
people, of course, is whether or not particular patterns of attributions
lead to more successful coping than others. Thus I was particularly
interested in finding out (1) whether chronically ill persons indeed
make attributions for their illness, (2) what attributions they make, and
(3) what attributions are most functional from a psychological
standpoint (e.g., help them cope better).

The ill all make attributions for their illness, as we can see from
the responses to the "why me?" question. As mentioned above, many
chronically ill people wondered whether the illness was a "punishment
from God" and were trying to figure out "why," since they felt it was
"undeserved punishment." As a respondent speculated, "It must

be—is just a part of my trials and tribulations God put upon me to make me stronger and to change me." Another person obviously thought that maybe it was "deserved punishment" or a test of some kind. He was more specific, wondering, "Why wasn't it my older brother? This is hereditary! My brother ought to have been the one who inherited this disease! However, there is a reason why I have this disease. . . . My goals used to be set on money and putting myself first; . . . now that this has come my way, it has changed my whole perspective and outlook on life. . . . It made me more aware of not putting material things ahead of God." In fact, a few respondents mentioned that it must be hereditary, naming some relatives that "probably" had the same or similar illness: "My mother and her mother before her also suffered from these damn chronic headaches! So, what can be done about it? Not a thing!"

A few others attributed their illness to their family's lifestyle, especially to their family's eating habits. As a respondent recalled with mixed emotions,

> When you get hit like this, and you start to do a little reading, then I can look in that respect and I can see where—this is not to criticize my parents, but the way I was brought up and the type of food that we had—there was a lot of rich apple pie, and roast beef and gravy and—Basically, I held a stable diet of meat and fish, chicken, turkey, everything. My mother was a fabulous cook! Everything was rich, rich, rich! So, from a dietary perspective, everything was done the wrong way.

Another respondent attributed her current heart problems to her parents' ignorance, and negligence, or rather to their well-meaning, but too permissive child-rearing practices:

> [I had] a mild case of strep, and it was undiagnosed and untreated and the heart thing showed up later . . . somewhere along the line. And in fact, I can remember a time in seventh or eighth grade when I had a really bad sore throat. . . . A particular doctor always gave me a penicillin shot. You walk in his office and you got a penicillin shot, and I didn't want that! So, whether or not it was my fault, and my parents didn't know anything about strep throats and watching out for that, so that's the only thing I can begin to relate to it. . . . My parents felt real guilty about it.

They think that it was from that fever, that maybe they should have recognized that something was wrong with me and they didn't. Although they never expressed that to me, I think I can tell. My father in particular!

Some chronically ill people talked about family or occupational stress being the probable cause of their illness. For example, a man attributed his heart condition to the aggravations cause by the "constant bickering at home by my children—two teenage daughters and a 27-year-old son who still lives at home with a very bad attitude, expecting everybody to wait on him, . . . and to the responsibilities of running the household."

Another respondent attributed the exacerbations of her illness symptoms and most of her secondary health problems to stressful conditions at work:

I was going to college, everything was still quiet, things were coming one thing at a time, the stress I had was positive. I got down working at Illinois Bell and the whole life turned around. I went from a very quiet childhood and young adulthood into mass production with corporate structure, and I've had to—at the time I didn't realize I had to do this, but now, looking back, it's easier to understand. I had to go into being a person that had to make a lot of decisions for a lot of people and—Did I have a responsible position? Very responsible! Very stressful! Constant stress! It got to the point, the last four years I worked at Illinois Bell, I think, . . . part of that made me realize that I'm stepping out of my boundaries. The responsibility got to the point where I had less and less time to take care of my basic health. I forgot. One could easily forget when things are going well. I have this thing that needs time and I've had these other things that, you know, you look and say, You have to earn your living, you have to function, and you want to function actually better than a normal person because you want people to look at you and say, Wow! She can handle it. She's qualified. Don't even bring up the diabetes unless it has to be brought up. You don't want to sit and say I can't function because I have this.

As I had hypothesized, for most people, becoming chronically ill does inevitably seem to lead to concentrated efforts in self-examination and social perception, through engaging in the attributional process. Since I had initially made that assumption, I also wondered what attributions would be most functional from a psychological standpoint. In other words, if people attribute their illness to chance or to the environment (external causes) versus to themselves (internal causes), do they perceive themselves as having less control over the course of their illness? If so, which type of belief would lead to better coping with and/or managing the illness? Furthermore, in what kinds of behaviors does the perception of control manifest itself?

The general concept of "locus of control" refers to the belief that events are either internally or externally controlled. "Health locus of control," developed and tested by Richard Lau (1982), is a more specific form of this concept, referring to people's beliefs that they can exert control over their state of health (an internal health locus of control) or that prevention of illness is beyond their control (external health locus of control).

A number of studies show that internal locus of control, defined as the perception of oneself as to some degree able to affect the course of the illness, is an asset in positive adjustment; that is, it is associated with more constructive responses. Kobasa (1982, p. 3) suggests that "control allows persons to perceive many stressful life events as predictable consequences of their own activity and, thereby, as subject to their direction and manipulation." This pattern suggests that internal locus of control is strongly related to long-term adjustment.

Furthermore, the importance of psychological control emerges not only in the attribution of causes for a negative event such as discovering one has an incurable illness, but also in how these people approach their follow-up care. For people who are victimized by an incurable illness, this issue of psychological control raises the conceptual importance of distinguishing between responsibility for initial causes and responsibility for solutions.

As a matter of fact, in recent years, social psychologists have become increasingly interested in the issue of victimization. Various theorists have suggested that reactions to victimization may be affected by such motives as (1) the desire to maintain a belief in a "just world," in which people have a need to believe that victims get what they deserve and deserve what they get (Lerner 1965, 1971; Lerner & Matthews 1967; Lerner & Simmons 1966); (2) the desire to protect oneself from blame in order to maintain or enhance one's self-esteem, termed "defensive attribution" (Shaver 1970); and (3) the desire to maintain a belief that one is in control over one's own fate, in which blame is assigned to someone else possibly responsible for the event or causality is assigned to an unpredictable, uncontrollable set of circumstances when the consequences of the event become increasingly severe (Kelley 1971; Walster 1966). In this way, individuals can either reassure themselves that they will be able to avoid similar disasters or, in some cases, are forced to concede that such events might happen to them again.

The emphasis on the desire for control has been treated more systematically by Kelley (1971, p. 22), who suggests that "attribution processes are to be understood not only as a means of providing the individual with a veridical view of his world, but as a means of encouraging and maintaining his effective exercise of control in that world." Hence, it follows that defensive attribution theorists would predict that people would ascribe their suffering to external factors rather than to their own shortcomings, presumably to maintain a positive self-view. Neither Walster nor Kelley, however, in their concern with control, have specifically discussed how this motive might affect the attributions of those victimized by misfortune themselves. The motive to maintain a positive self-view could lead an individual to blame those factors that are most within that individual's control. In other words, victims would be most apt to attribute blame to their own behaviors only if these behaviors were easily modifiable. If these people were unable or unwilling to change their behaviors, blame would be ascribed to external factors. Thus it stands to reason that attributions would be made to external factors, because they are the most elusive and uncontrollable of factors.

Although the evidence is far from conclusive, it is interesting to note that, with the exception of two persons, none of my respondents blamed themselves for their misfortune. One respondent felt that she possibly brought her diabetes on herself by being a "sweetoholic" and claimed that she has since greatly modified her eating habits. The other respondent, who attributed his illness as possible punishment for being selfish and too materialistic, also said that he has since changed his priorities and behavior. I might add, at the risk of sounding cynical, that if indeed these people changed their behaviors as they claimed, there was not much else they could have done anyway under their particular circumstances. And, virtually nobody else attributed

illness to him- or herself (e.g., to self-initiated behaviors), not even
the "heavy smoker" or the person who admitted having "a drinking
problem in the past," although there are illnesses known to be affected
by these habits, as in the relation between smoking and heart disease
or lung cancer and emphysema.

Two other respondents, male and female, both highly educated
people, simply attributed their illness to chance, also an external
factor: The first respondent said, "Why me? That's an easy question.
An easy question! In the scheme of things, in the scheme of the
universe and the scheme of the whole thing, me is an unimportant — It
happened to me like it would to anyone else, and I don't ask the
question, Why me? I just accept it as a part of my place. I figured it
could've happened to anybody else. . . . I look at it in that respect."
The second respondent said, "Why me? Oh! It's just luck, bad luck!"

In short, chronically ill respondents mostly attributed their illness,
one way or another, to external factors, including to "aging" and plain
"bad luck." In retrospect, this should not have been surprising, since
attribution research reveals that good outcomes are attributed to
oneself much more than are bad outcomes.

At first, I had thought that there might be quite a few people who
would believe that maybe they deserved their illness because of their
past behaviors or lifestyles (e.g., smoking, drinking, and improper
diet). Thus I had also speculated that if chronically ill people came to
believe that they deserved the outcomes they received, they would
blame or derogate themselves, and thus they might resign themselves
to their fate and become passive sufferers.

On the contrary, I found that, faced with an incurable and progressive illness, most chronically ill people interviewed responded in
surprisingly hopeful terms. They adopted specific strategies to
convince themselves and others around them that they were not
responsible for their misfortune and that they were not helpless
victims, but rather in control of their situation.

Some chronically ill people went even further and evaluated the
unfortunate situation as a positive event and expressed the sentiments
that the illness had a positive overall influence on their lives (e.g.,
made them better persons). As a respondent explained, "You begin
to get in tune with things. . . . It gives you a level of understanding
and along with this thing a kind of peace of mind. . . . It makes you
a little more sensitive; by sensitive I don't mean a touchy form. I

mean sensitive for recognizing stuff, appreciating the thing. . . . You have to be sensitive to appreciate people." Another person thought that the illness made him more health conscious in a preventative sense: "When you pay attention to your medical condition, you know, you go to a doctor more frequently, so if there's anything, you can catch it in the beginning."

The strategies employed by these people to convince themselves and others that they are in control of their situations and/or that they are actually receiving some benefit from their misfortunes are strategies clearly designed to maintain or renew a positive perception of the self. Thus, contrary to a generalized public perception that chronically ill persons are on a hopeless, downward trajectory, my data indicate that coping with chronic illness is an active and resourceful process.

In fact, I found that a surprising number of chronically ill persons saw their illness as a challenge to be conquered, a war to be won, probably because this perspective seems to give them a sense of control. There seems to be a sense of accomplishment and pride in defeating the odds, as one of my respondents declared: "I outlived — The doctors can't believe I'm still alive. I've outlived the curve! I don't know if you know about the curve of open heart surgery? Well, there's no absolute, but I had eight years after the first one, '70 to '78. I never expected to reach age sixty-five! I never expected to reach age sixty-six!"

Furthermore, many people "personified" the illness and gave it personal qualities. They talked about being invaded by this foreign enemy to whom they were not going to give in. This phenomenon is also expressed in a popular television commercial that says, "I have arthritis but arthritis does not have me." Indeed, these chronically ill persons were particularly proud of how they were "winning" and were able to manage their very difficult circumstances. This response was particularly true of younger respondents:

> I never wanted to accept the problem. I'm trying to fight it. I fight it by staying active in sports. . . . When I play baseball I believe that I am Ryne Sandberg! . . . I can't view myself being pushed around in a wheelchair by my wife and daughter. . . . I have a strong will power.

However, older chronic sufferers do not seem to be as hopeful; the attribution process especially creates problems for them. Indeed, there is a general tendency in our culture to over-attribute all negative changes in health and mood to aging per se, especially to the presumed physical decline associated with aging, thereby incorrectly focusing the person away from stress-inducing situational and social factors that may affect health. For example, a 50-year-old respondent stated, "Well, I just don't feel like I was 20 anymore. I feel like I'm old, not ancient, but old. When I was young I didn't have no problems with arthritis. I mean I did, but it never bothered me. But now that I got arthritis, I feel like I'm getting old." A 53-year-old respondent, a woman who suffers from not one but three chronic conditions (epilepsy, diabetes, and heart problems), still attributed her many physical symptoms to aging, rather than to the illnesses. In fact, she seemed to be comfortable with the notion that people are likely to get these illnesses as they get older: "You know, when you get older, some of these things happen. Yeah, I know!"

Many health care professionals, including physicians and nurses, also assume that a certain amount of limiting illness is normal for an aging person, an assumption that is absolutely untrue. According to Atchley (1985), although limiting chronic conditions are common among older people, many of these conditions are preventable, most are treatable, and all can be successfully managed to some extent if they are perceived as atypical at any age, rather than normal for older people. Thus, when events are attributed to the aging process and are seen as inevitable, remedial steps, that could be extremely beneficial are not undertaken. As another one of my respondents, a 52-year-old woman who is suffering daily from all sorts of bodily pains she attributes to "probably having arthritis," perceived by her as a natural consequence of aging, said, "What can the doctors do? When you're getting older, the body falls apart. . . . So, I don't even bother anymore, I take my aspirins or whatever will help and I do what I have to do."

The influence of age on responses to chronic illness must be further investigated. So far the research results have been contradictory. There is evidence, for instance, that older persons become more disabled by the same diseases than younger persons (Haber 1971). On the other hand, Singer (1974) found that younger persons afflicted with Parkinson's disease were more upset and disabled than older patients.

Clearly, then, it is necessary to separate the effects people attribute to the aging process from those they attribute to their chronic illness. This separation might be accomplished by research using a more diverse sample (e.g., people of different age groups afflicted with the same illness), as I have attempted to do in choosing my respondents for this study.

My findings indicate that older persons do indeed attribute many of their problems to aging, and in many cases they are reinforced in these beliefs by their families, friends, and health care professionals. Even when some of them try to figure out cause-and-effect relationships and rationally attribute their symptoms to illness conditions rather than to aging, these people report that they are often discouraged and even derogated by those around them. "What do you expect? You are getting older" is a very common reply to their concerns. For example, a 55-year-old respondent related that when he tried to discuss with his doctor his symptoms and his limitations, particularly the fact that he was not able to do certain things he was always able to do, he was cut short and given the following explanation by his doctor: "You're not 18 years old."

Younger persons, in particular, seem to feel rather cheated by having a chronic illness. In line with the general cultural belief, some of them mentioned that they thought "only older people are supposed to get such an illness," and thus these younger sufferers seem to resent the illness, rebel against it, and try much harder not to give in to the "sick role."

Although I do not have extensive and conclusive data to support my claim, I still came to the conclusion, similar to that of Taylor, Lichtman, and Wood (1984), that regardless of what people, young or old, attribute their illness to, the rate at which these individuals recover from major surgery or adequately adapt to living a fairly normal life with illness conditions seems to be influenced by their beliefs about the possibility of exercising some control over their future condition—control exercised either by themselves or by a physician.

What happens to people when they cannot control their condition? In fact, I wondered what happens to people when they repeatedly experience negative outcomes, for example, discover that they cannot control the progressive deterioration of their illness despite all their positive efforts (e.g., strictly following regimens). Do they give up? Does "learned helplessness" set in?

My findings, in line with victimization studies, indicate that although enhanced feelings of personal control may generally be adaptive, they are maladaptive when individuals are confronted with permanent, nonmodifiable outcomes; in other words, their efforts toward adaptation do not work when they become victims of uncontrollable circumstances.

In fact, my data indicate that the more "independent" people perceive themselves to be, the harder it is for them to adapt to illness conditions and to accept the limitations imposed by these conditions. Their actual age does not seem to be as important a factor in this process as their perception of themselves. In other words, people who view them-selves as independent, no matter how old, try to normalize their lives as much as possible in spite of their limitations, often at the expense of their health. Their efforts at normalization are directed mostly at countering the effects of uncertainty and stigma, the most problematic characteristics of chronic illness, and avoiding social isolation—the major consequence.

1

Uncertainty: A Key Characteristic of Chronic Illness

The course of events is unpredictable in chronic illness, in which remissions and exacerbations occur. In fact, chronic illness has been described by Wiener (1975) as an experience of living with chronic uncertainty. Uncertainty does not represent the total experience of chronic illness, yet it is a constant and most problematic part of it. Thus, the concept of uncertainty must be addressed in order to understand the problematic nature of chronic illnesses. Uncertainty, is defined as the inability to determine the meaning of events, occurs in a situation where the decision-maker is unable to assign definite values to objects and events and/or is unable to predict outcomes accurately.

In the illness experience, uncertainty arises when (1) people lack information about the diagnosis and seriousness of their illness (2) they cannot make predictions as to the course of the illness and its prognosis (3) they have ambiguity concerning the stage of their illness (e.g., how advanced it is), and (4) they lack information regarding the best and/or alternate treatments and systems of care.

Strauss and colleagues (1975; 1984) used the term "trajectory" in their discussion of the uncertainty of chronic illness. They coined the term "illness trajectory" to refer not only to the physiological manifestations of a sick person's disease but also to the "total organization of work done over that course, plus the impact on those involved with that work and its organization" (1984, p. 64). They noted that uncertain courses of illness and illness trajectories tend to maximize personal and familial hardships.

When I asked my respondents to describe the most problematic aspect of their illness, the concept of uncertainty emerged as the most salient problematic characteristic of chronic illness. Uncertainty did not start out as a major focus of my research, but it turned out to be the aspect of chronic illness that seems most to affect the adaptation versus normalization processes of ill people, because it undermines their quality of life.

Koocher (1984) reports that uncertainty regarding the duration of an illness or its oucome is the greatest single psychological stressor for people with life-threatening chronic illness. Although the outcome may not be the desired choice, knowledge of it is preferable because it removes the uncertainty. Many researchers (Mishel et al. 1984; Richardson et al. 1987; Hilton 1988; Webster & Christman 1988; Wineman 1990), found that uncertainty led to anxiety and depression. Most respondents reported the experience of uncertainty as emotionally painful.

Certain illnesses and their possible developments are well known, as is the impact of their treatments. For these illnesses the course of illness is fairly predictable; their phases and the relative rate at which the phases will change can be more or less anticipated. When symptoms form a pattern, less uncertainty and less ambiguity exist about the state of the illness, so ill people have a clearer appraisal of their disease state and can monitor their progress and the effectiveness of their treatments (e.g., a diabetic patient can periodically test her or his blood sugar levels).

For other illnesses, such as multiple sclerosis, epilepsy, lupus, Crohn's disease, and rheumatoid arthritis, both the phases and their rates of change are very uncertain. A major characteristic of many of these illnesses is not that they are curable or incurable, but that their manifestations and trajectories are unpredictable and the management methods for them are uncertain. These illnesses do not follow a strictly downhill course. Flare-ups occur suddenly, and in some cases, they can also be suddenly arrested; their trajectories can be quite calm for a long time, only to burst out again. People complain that they do not know what type of symptoms will occur (i.e., pain, stiffness, swelling, and numbness), where on their body they will occur, how severe they will be, or how long they will last. Some respondents reported that never know from one day to the next how sick they will be. But even with relatively predictable illnesses, the sequential phases do not appear and disappear in a definite time pattern. This matter of uncertainty is of utmost importance, because the efficiency of treatments and social arrangements are closely linked with the predictability of the trajectories.

Problems in family relationships have been reported as resulting from uncertainty (Mishel et al. 1984; Rowat & Knafl 1985). Uncertainty can affect day-to-day functioning by sabotaging adjustments in the major areas of family, work, and recreation, because the family's day-to-day living becomes indeterminate. For example, people suffering from rheumatoid arthritis find planning ahead impossible owing to unexpected pain and stiffness. Lazarus (1974) suggested that when an event such as chronic illness has an uncertain outcome, it is judged to be a serious threat, because the person is not able to get a clear idea of what is to occur. Shalitt (1977) stated that the ambiguity factor in uncertainty has the highest threat potential because it makes locating hazardous situations difficult and thus impedes effective coping. A respondent who thought that she could control her illness by avoiding potentially harmful activities and situations, yet still found herself in trouble, explained: "I could just be sitting at home doing absolutely nothing and all of a sudden, I'll start having trouble breathing. It happened to me one time when I was sitting at home watching television, and all of a sudden I started feeling like I couldn't breathe. It could've been for any number of reasons, but – "

Mishel (1981) also noted that uncertainty hampers the formation of a plan of action, limiting individuals' abilities to evaluate their situation adequately, and according to Mishel and Sorenson (1991), it also weakens their sense of mastery over a situation. Murdaugh and Mishel (1991), found that uncertainty weakens internal locus of control; Braden (1990) reported that uncertainty reduced their sense of learned resourcefulness among chronically ill persons suffering from

rheumatoid arthritis, which in turn lessened their ability to help themselves.

Indeed, we know from the social psychological literature that
individuals define situations through some cognitive process and that,
based on this evaluation, they determine the appropriate management
strategies (Lazarus 1966; Mechanic 1974; Chirisman 1977; Lazarus &
Cohen 1977; Shalit 1977). A major and erroneous assumption made
in most discussions of cognitive evaluation, however, is that the
person in question has complete information about the situation being
appraised. On the contrary, in most cases of chronic illness, there is
considerable uncertainty and lack of information. For instance, the
symptoms of a disease, although routinely seen by physicians and
known to them to be non-life-threatening, may nevertheless be
unfamiliar, unexpected, confusing, and frightening to patients.
Physicians who tell patients to relax, not to worry, to reduce their
activities, or to call back later if the symptoms persist — commonly
known as the "take two aspirins and call me in the morning diagnosis" — without giving any explanations for these symptoms or any
rationale for their advice only add to the uncertainty and fear that most
of these patients feel. A respondent, recalling a very frightening
experience, said:

> I was having an attack at the time. The first thing he did was give
> me a shot in the arm. You know, I just asked him, I go, "What
> exactly is going on?" He goes, "You have asthma!" He didn't
> really say much. He didn't tell me that much. He just gave me a
> shot and told me to go get a prescription filled, and that was about
> it. And I'm not even sure if he gave me a pamphlet on it. . . . He
> just told me that I have it and that's about it.

There is a certain amount of uncertainty and stress inherent in
living with a chronic illness, but when people have to make their
decisions on the basis of limited or incorrect information, this creates
additional and unnecessary uncertainty and stress, making a difficult
situation even worse. Chronically ill people, like most of us, are not
experts in the health care field. Further, they are usually given limited
or no information about their illness, and its treatment methods and
alternatives by those who treat them, under the assumption that these
ill people would not be able to comprehend all these complex issues.
Thus these chronically ill people have to make crucial decisions

affecting all aspects of their lives based on insufficient information, at a time when they are most vulnerable and anxious. Therefore, providing chronically ill persons with sufficient information about their illness and available treatment alternatives is one important means of reducing the uncertainty, the stress, and the need to search for causal explanations that they all experience. Lack of confidence and trust in the physician results in high levels of uncertainty. Mishel (1988) found that confidence and trust in the physician explained 35 percent of the variance in uncertainty, because the physician is a source of information about causes and consequences of symptoms. The more credible the physician, the less the uncertainty.

When events are recognized as familiar, less uncertainty exists about the complexity of treatment and the system of care. Knowledge of the usual symptom display allows the sufferer a degree of control because it allows comparisons for monitoring changes during treatment. Direct inquiry by health care providers to elicit sufferers' concerns about their illness and response to these concerns improves their understanding of the symptom pattern. Thus effective communication between health care providers and the chronically ill about the causes and consequences of symptoms serves to alleviate some uncertainty and fear and can be an important factor in determining the way ill persons evaluate their situations. As one respondent stated:

> Some people might not be happy with a doctor that will tell you every thing; my doctor will, and he's been very supportive; he's honest. He tells you there is no miracle cure for it; . . . he says if you have any questions about it, just ask me, and I'll find out any answers that are available. Matter of fact, the last time I saw him he gave me a book he wanted me to look over. I explained to him, I said, well — he realized I can't read too well — so I says what will happen is my wife will read it to me. I picked out a chapter that I was interested in at the time and my wife read the whole book. . . . He said let him know what you guys think of it, and we told him that we thought it was a fairly good description of it and it didn't hold anything back.

In fact, persons who recently have been diagnosed as having a long-term chronic illness are profoundly fearful and uncertain about many things. An environment that was formerly at least tolerable has now become unpredictable and threatening, bringing the former assumptions and beliefs these persons have about the self and the environment into question. These people are thus confronted with a web of fears, including fear of pain, of recurrence, of progressive deterioration, of dying, and, most likely, of dependency on medications and other people. A respondent expressed these feelings: "I don't want to be dependent on it, you know, I can't see myself doing that for the rest of my life, although I know someone with asthma, it's very possible. My uncle had asthma and he was dependent on medication for all of his life, but I don't like to be dependent on things, or on people either. Not too much."

Most people also worry about whether the doctors have been honest with them, whether they are receiving the best care available, and how their illness will affect their families, friendships, and work situations. The respondent just quoted was fighting against dependency on medications but was forced to give in because she was worried about her relationships, feeling even more reluctant to be dependent on other people than on medications.

> I kept having to stop and, you know, trying to catch my breath and go a few more feet and then stop because I didn't have the medicine to help me out. . . . I didn't want to have to put them through it. I'm like, I'm really sorry to be doing this to you guys and everything, 'cause they'd take me home and make sure that I was okay, so now I just always carry it [the medicine] with me. So, I guess I'm not so much a burden to everyone else.

These people are forced to contend with a variety of physical changes and problems, which may include pain, disfigurement, nausea, energy loss, and malodors. Clearly such changes are deeply unsettling and can have a profound effect on persons' self-concepts, and consequently on their relationships. What is ironic is that within the context of this uncertainty about the changing environment and self, chronically ill individuals are often called upon to function more competently and more rationally than ever before in making the many decisions that confront them. These decisions range from questions about which physician to contact, what hospital to enter, and what treatment to have to questions about what to tell spouses, children, friends, and co-workers. Thus, most ill people are at first over-whelmed by the number and complexity of decisions to be made.

While these decisions are similar to those that people make in everyday life, they are linked to graver consequences, and chronically ill persons are emotionally and physically less able to tackle them. In addition, a large number of these decisions concern matters with which most people have no prior expertise or experience. The respondent just mentioned, finally realizing how intrusive her illness really was, said, "It's really strange, cause like, you know, when they said I had asthma, I never thought of that as really a chronic illness, but you know, I guess it is! I don't usually think about it that much. I just cope with it from day to day. I just make the best of it I can."

As a matter of fact, there is considerable ambiguity within the field of medicine itself about how to treat many chronic conditions, since most of them, by definition, cannot be cured at this stage of our medical knowledge. Unlike the case of acute illness, medicine has made little progress in the treatment of chronic illness, which is not susceptible to a single-cause approach. As far as we know, at this state of our knowledge, many chronic illnesses seem to have no known physical cause. Consequently, as mentioned in the introductory chapter, the rise and prevalance of chronic illness has led to the development of multicausal theories of disease, including theories relating to differences in lifestyles and socioenvironmental stress in causation of disease. Unfortunately, there may be no clear-cut answers to some of the problems facing afflicted individuals.

The literature pertinent to how physicians deal with uncertainty has received increasing attention in recent years (Bosk 1979; Fox 1980; Light 1980). First explored by Renee C. Fox (1957), this dimension of medical training creates a double bind for physicians. Uncertainty pervades their work and they must be open to it yet their license and mandate from society presumes they know how to take care of problems that ordinary persons are uncertain how to address. It is interesting to note that Oliver Wendell Holmes wrote to a young physician, "Let me recommend to you, as far as possible, to keep your doubts to yourself, and give the patient the benefit of your decision" (quoted in Mumford 1970, p. 163). Indeed, there is a lot of evidence in the health and illness literature focusing on doctor-patient relationships that this advice is well followed. For instance, until recently, patients were not even allowed to see their own charts, and most of the time, they still do not have access to vital information about their conditions. When patients ask to see their charts, they are, frequently met with suspicion and hostility, because the assumption is made that they are gathering material to bring legal action against their doctors or the hospital.

Whatever the reason, most of the time, ill persons are not told about treatment alternatives. For instance, some surgeons are still performing mastectomies when in fact many studies in the last 20 years have demonstrated that less disfiguring procedures, such as removing only the malignant lesion and radiotherapy, produce the same survival rates as removing the whole breast, a procedure that can have devastating psychological effects on some women. As another example, there are almost as many different kinds of operations for treating heart conditions as there are prominent heart surgeons in our society. Some of these procedures are less debilitating, yet seem to show the same survival rates as the more drastic measures. But since chronically ill persons are not usually informed about all the different kinds of operations available, it is often impossible for them to feel confident that the chosen treatments are the best ones. One of my respondents, who had been a general practitioner for over twenty years before he "suddenly collapsed into a coma because of kidney failure" and found himself a reluctant "patient," exclaimed, "I never realized what patients have to go through! It's been quite an education. They treat you like morons, they come and go, do things to you, and they don't tell you anything. Yes, even me!" In fact, people customarily get the treatments their particular physician or surgeon is trained in or familiar with, and are not fully informed about alternative procedures, regardless of their effectiveness or cost.

Of course, there are many reasons why physicians might communicate in a manner that leaves patients confused and frustrated: (1) they might not know exactly what to do or be able to predict outcome, (2) the known treatments may have been exhausted with no positive results, or (3) as a result of treating some symptoms, additional and unexpected problems ("iatrogenic diseases") may arise.

Fox (1989) notes that:

the mode of thought on which modern medical science and research are based is an emergent, eclectic product of the numerous fields of biological, physical, and behavioral science on which it draws. Biology is its cornerstone, but the phenomena with which medicine deals are both too complex and too individuated to be confined to a purely biological analysis, or to any single explanatory theory. (p. 183)

She further notes that:

by its very nature, . . . scientific research is fraught with uncertainty, with seemingly aleatory events, and with limitations in knowledge—including those that are inherent to scientific ways of knowing. . . . Medical researchers experience these problems in a particularly acute and often painful way. They are faced with the immediate consequences for health and illness, life and death, of what they do not know or understand, and cannot control. (p. 183)

Indeed, doctors complain that they never expected the degree of uncertainty inherent in medicine when they chose it as a career and that they have problems dealing with the stress the uncertainty exerts.

In her earlier research, Fox (1959) has documented the agony of well-intentioned and sincere physicians who vigorously treat disease only to find that the treatment itself creates unresolvable complications, seen as medical failures by patients and physicians alike. Indeed, failure is difficult to acknowledge by anyone, and telling patients and their families that nothing more can be done cannot be easy.

How do patients deal with uncertainty? I thought that one of the most fascinating questions about the chronically ill had to be how they evaluate their own adjustment to their condition. Indeed, because of the uncertainties they face and because their sense of self is threatened, many chronically ill persons probably experience intense needs both to clarify what is happening to them and to be supported and reassured by others. Thus, I hypothesized that if people think they are dealing badly with their illness, such thinking will be an added strain on what may be an already difficult existence, whereas if these individuals feel they are adjusting well, that belief can be a source of satisfaction and pride.

As Schachter (1959) stated, people often seek out other people for purposes of social comparison or reassurance when doubts arise about their own experiences. As far as chronic illness is concerned, this process of social comparison, although essential, can have serious consequences at times, because some people might exacerbate a problem by persisting in behaviors condoned or encouraged by others; they might postpone treatment until it is too late, having been told by others that treatment is either hopeless or unnecessary, or they might discontinue an effective therapy, impressed by the negative reactions of their families and friends.

Whatever the consequences, chronically ill people, like all individuals, do indeed compare themselves to others, yet they do it somewhat differently. The literature on social comparison demonstrates that in general individuals compare themselves with people who are doing slightly better than they are. According to Festinger (1954), although one comes off as psychologically disadvantaged, one may gain useful information from the upward comparison.

There are indications, however, that some people, including chronically ill people, appear instead to be making downward comparisons, so they come off as somewhat psychologically advantaged and informed. Some research on social comparison indicates that this pattern of downward comparison is particularly likely to occur under conditions of threat (Hakmiller 1966; Wheeler et al. 1969). This finding might suggest that these individuals may be selecting their comparisons to preserve their self-esteem rather than letting self-esteem be determined by those readily available for comparison. Such downward comparisons as "I'm really much better off than she/he is" can bolster peoples' own sense of self, and might convince them that they are adapting well to their difficult circumstances.

My data strongly support this finding; of all the people I interviewed, not a single person seemed to know anybody suffering from the same illness who was better off than themselves. These people either said they knew of no one in the same circumstances or told me horror stories about similar cases. For example, when asked if she knew other people with the same illness, a respondent replied by recalling a certain event:

> My brother-in-law got married, and his wife's father had MS. I never met the man because he was bedridden in the hospital in Park Forest. In Park Forest? I never could keep them straight, out south somewhere, but they never said too much about him. I just was always like, well, why couldn't he come to the wedding? At least, they could have done that for him. But at the time I didn't realize he was so bad. They just couldn't put him in a wheelchair

and bring him to the wedding. Ya know, when you first get these things, and you don't wind up flat on your back, you don't realize what the worst is.

It seems, for reasons of reassurance and/or preservation of self-esteem, chronically ill people often look to people in similar circumstances to gather information about and evaluate their conditions, their feelings, and their behaviors in order to reduce their illness-related uncertainties and, particularly, in order to evaluate their own performances. But to bolster their self-esteem and make themselves feel and look good, they seem to select or remember only "worst scenario" examples and thus to compare themselves only to people who are worse off than themselves. On closer examination, this phenomenon turns out to be an important normalization strategy.

In short, the problem of uncertainty for people with chronic illnesses is recognized, but few studies have addressed this most important issue. As Parsons (1951) noted, distress or at least uneasiness with the uncertainty inherent in chronic illness is to be expected in a society that emphasizes what he called "mastery" of health. My data show that chronically ill people use various behavioral and cognitive strategies to deal with or sidestep the issue of uncertainty.

2

The Stigma of Chronic Illness

According to Jennings, Callahan, and Caplan (1988, p. 6), "Chronic illness and disability are often stigmatizing; intolerance, fear, and misunderstanding, at one extreme, and well meaning but humiliating and patronizing sympathy at the other often greet the chronically ill in their everyday social lives."

In our society, as in most, any illness is negatively valued, and noncurable long-term illnesses are particularly problematic. Parsons (1951) appropriately summarized the American expectation regarding health by noting that the society asserts the desirability of mastery of the problems of health. Parsons stated that the concept of health is particularly salient in American society because of the society's value system, which emphasizes independence and individual achievement, and the high level of differentiation in its social structure. Parsons (1972, 1975) suggested that illness is dysfunctional to the social system because it hinders individuals and weakens their effective performance of social roles. He said that society views illness as a form of deviance that needs to be controlled because it poses problems both for the individual and society. Parsons (1951) stated that persons who are ill are allowed certain exemptions and privileges denied to other types of social deviants. But at the same time, these individuals acquire certain obligations, suggesting that the person who assumes the "sick role" has to deal with four institutionalized expectations and obligations: (1) the sick person is exempt from normal social role responsibilities, (2) the sick person is not held responsible for the illness and cannot become well purely by an act of will, (3) the state of being ill is undesirable and carries an obligation to get well, and (4) the sick person is obligated to seek technically competent help and to cooperate with that help to achieve a speedy recovery.

From Parsons's (1951) perspective, sickness is a temporary deviant role the individual plays to deal with a particular problem while trying to return to a healthy, normal-functioning state. Thus the sick role ideally, and almost perfectly, fits acute illnesses and temporary disabilities caused by accidents. The members of society tolerate such short-term deviance since it is understandable, can happen to anyone, and, in the long run, is beneficial for the group, but must be legitimated and controlled.

As an ideal model, Parsons's sick role concept has been widely analyzed, applied, and criticized—mostly for its limited applicability to people with chronic conditions (Cogswell & Weir 1973; Kassenbaum & Baumann 1965; Callahan et al. 1966; Levine & Kozloff 1978), and mainly because sick persons do not get well from most chronic conditions and some acute ones (e.g., polio). Instead, the disease process may be arrested in such a manner that the affected individuals are considered to be well, yet either continuous treatment is needed to forestall death (e.g., diabetes, renal failure) or permanent residual damage remains because of the disease process (e.g., paralysis from polio). From the perspective of societal standards, such persons are incapacitated (deviant) to some degree, and at the same time they must define the new capacity level as normal for them and find ways to continue performing their role obligations, since their conditions are permanent. Thus, both the normal expectations for well people and the special expectations for sick people would be considered inappropriate. In short, chronically ill people find themselves in "no-win" situations.

Gordon (1966) tried to apply Parsons's sick role model to a variety of chronic conditions, and found that the expectations held for people of this type could be described in terms of an "impaired role." The impaired role parallels the sick role, with the exception that people are not exempt from normal activities but rather are expected to engage in them as much as possible within the limits of their impairment. A respondent, addressing this issue, gave a couple of examples:

> Like, we used to have a dirt floor in our basement, you know, and my father would say: well, why don't you go down and clean it, not thinking that, that would have some effect on my asthma . . . I can't go quite as fast and do some of the things they want me to do as quickly, or a lot of times they'll be doing some heavy moving or something and I will just tell them: you guys have to slow down. . . . I think my friends are closer than my family. My friends will slow down, you know, if I need them to without me saying anything. But my family, you know, like they expect you to pull your share, and if you can't, you have to say something.

The whole concept of "normalization" speaks to this phenomenon. Chronically ill people are indeed expected to fulfill their duties and obligations in their families like everybody else, and because they are aware of this expectation, some of these people, using self-presentational tactics and many other strategies, try very hard to carry on with their usual activities, even at the expense of their health.

Although Parsons's sick role model may not apply to chronic illnesses as perfectly as it applies to acute illnesses, his perception of illness as a deviant state is even more important to the study of chronic illness than it is to the examination of acute illness. As Parsons (1951) so perceptively suggested, to be sick or to have a disorder is to go through something unfortunate, bad, or undesirable.

Furthermore, the metaphor of illness (Sontag 1978, 1989) also conveys strangeness, victimization, pity, and in some cases even revulsion. Sontag (1978, 1989) suggested that any disease that is treated as a mystery because of unknown etiology and is thus intensely feared will be felt to be morally, if not literally, contagious. This moral component of illness is most apparent in the chronic conditions in which distinctions between disease or disorder and self become blurred. A passing cold, flu, or even a more serious acute condition do not have the implications for self or identity that chronic conditions do, because they are common temporary states leaving no residual disabilities and no permanent deviance. Chronic illness, on the other hand, threatens to leave a permanent stigma.

Freidson (1965) addressed the question of how a health state can become deviant, giving much significance to the legitimacy of stigma in illness. He suggested that if a stigma is attached to an illness, it also damages the ill person's identity and interferes with normal interaction, because while people may not hold ill persons responsible for their stigmatized condition, they are nonetheless upset, embarrassed or sometimes even revolted by it. One of my respondents mentioned that:

> There is lots of times that people don't know what to say to you. They come up with some weird things: Oh! You're looking good, or, You just look terrific. All positive things; they don't know how to come up and say, Well, what happened on your surgery? What did they have to do? Or, I would like them to ask me, How do you feel about having one breast off and one on? My daughter, she is a little scared and maybe a little embarrassed too, so I told her to tell people that her mother, she had a lump and it wasn't cancer.

When others become aware of a person's stigmatizing condition, they often react negatively, and the interaction or relationship between people becomes derailed. The stigmatizing condition often also leads to negative inferences about the person's abilities, characteristics, personality, and desirability. The condition becomes a stigma, and the person is said to be stigmatized. People not only evaluate stigmatized persons unfavorably, but they also behave differently toward them.

The Albrecht, Walker, and Levy (1982) study supported the view that most individuals place social distance between themselves and those with stigmatizing conditions because of ambiguity surrounding social interaction with such individuals. Ambiguity occurs, according to Preston (1979), when an individual encounters an element that does not fall within a specified range of normal variations and there is no alternate typification to account for the diversion. The incongruence is the source of ambiguity.

Preston's concept of ambiguity is closely related to Goffman's concept of stigma. Goffman (1963) defines stigma as the incongruence between the virtual social identity (the ideal) and the actual social identity (the real). In his classic book *Stigma: Notes on the Management of Spoiled Identity,* Erving Goffman (1963), addressed problems of the stigmatized individuals and suggested that the central feature in their situation is a question of acceptance. Handicapped and chronically ill persons share with many other people the problem of being stigmatized. That is, they have some characteristic that leads to a "spoiled identity, and renders the individual suspect in moral character." Goffman (1963) aptly noted that those who interact with stigmatized individuals focus primarily on the unacceptable differentness of these people, excluding traits considered normal. Goffman further noted that although not all handicapped persons suffer the visible impairments resulting in stigmatized identities, many suffer discreditation because of their decreased participation in the normal world. One respondent addressed this issue by noting that:

> I used to be like really afraid. I didn't want anyone to see that I was having problems breathing, that I had to take it [medicine], 'cause they'd always, you know, look at you, like, What are you doing? You know, are you taking drugs? . . . Why didn't I want them to know? I don't know. I guess, they would think you were different or, you know, . . . and I thought that maybe because I had asthma, that I wouldn't be exactly . . . part of the group.

These discredited definitions of self can arise in two ways: (1) in interaction with others and/or (2) out of unmet expectations of sick persons themselves. Among the most common reasons for discrediting by significant others is failure of the sick person to fulfill their expectations, whether or not these expectations are realistic. These expectations can range from performing simple household duties, work, and providing companionship to engaging in sexual activities.

Moreover, the situation can become worse for those people whose illnesses cause impairment, where the impairment remains relatively invisible. In these circumstances, others frequently pressure these ill people to remain functioning as before. Poor motivation tends to become the defined reason that they do not do so, rather than the person's physical condition (Siegler & Osmond 1979). Thus, chronically ill persons who cannot properly fulfill their obligations perceive that they are viewed in negative terms by those around them. They are accused of conspiring to get out of their obligations by performing poorly and functioning inadequately. As one respondent, a person who was becoming progressively blind from a condition that could not be corrected by glasses, recalled: "I was finally believed about my condition when I cracked up the family car against a wall I couldn't see and almost terminally injured myself. . . . I was trying to tell them I shouldn't be driving, I shouldn't go shopping. It was not taken seriously until then!"

Another respondent also addressed the issue of family expectations and pressure on chronically ill persons to function as before, regardless of their ability to do so, when she said:

> When you look at me, my whole household seems to be at a standstill, because I do everything. . . . When I married my husband, he used to do the chores, and when I quit working, I would do my own chores, and when I got sick, nobody did the chores, and I think that they didn't know to keep the household going without me, which irritated me more, and I would get frustrated 'cause I figured they're all grown, why do I? You know, and they can see how I can't lift. Why do they insist that I still make their dinner when I can't even lift a pan of water? And it would get to me that they're so inconsiderate, you know. And then, my doctor tried to tell me it's hard for them to cope with the change in you.

When ill persons realize that significant others do not understand or accept the limitations inherent in their present physical conditions, they feel discredited. As another example, a respondent mentioned that some people at her office repeatedly ask her if she wants coffee, rolls, or donuts, even though they know that she cannot have any because of her diabetes.

The most ordinary way that discrediting occurs is simply through being discounted or pitied, because being discounted is closely tied to the inability to function in conventional ways. The previous respondent also mentioned other occasions when people treat her as though she was abnormal or very sick simply because she could not eat certain foods or drink alcohol.

Being a "valid" person is a continual struggle for chronically ill people, and being "invalid" means acceptance of being discounted and devalued. Charmaz (1991, p. 109), notes that "chronically ill people wonder what they should tell and what they need to tell others about their conditions. . . . Telling often means exposing hidden feelings. Telling sometimes means straining relationships." She further notes that telling can also mean risking loss of control and acceptance for young and middle-aged adults, who can find themselves stigmatized and rejected or, at best, devalued and ignored. Older adults, especially single elderly women, risk losing their autonomy, their right to make decisions, their homes, their mobility, and their money, because adult children and/or service providers may assume they are not able to take care of themselves. When being discounted is constantly a threat, ill elderly people often feel compelled to negotiate their identities, even with family members. How successful they are in these negotiations certainly has great impact on their attempts to normalize their lives.

I can truly identify with what these respondents said because, although it was a long time ago, I still remember my own experiences as a young girl suffering from asthma. For example, I was always told by my parents, "If you can go to school, work, and go out with your friends, you can also contribute at home and clean house." My way of negotiating for my identity was to do what I was asked to do at home even though cleaning chores often resulted in exacerbations of my symptoms. My parents simply thought that I was trying to get out of work I disliked. I would try very hard to do these chores to avoid family arguments, but mostly to be able to participate in social activities with my friends without disclosing my illness to them. These activities were my attempts to normalize my life. I now realize that in order to avoid being stigmatized, I was also using many of the self-presentation tactics discussed later in this chapter. And because of my personal experience both as a person with a chronic condition and as a caregiver to my mother, I was able to identify and reach some insight into the normalization strategies used by chronically ill people as they arose in my respondents' descriptions of their daily living experiences.

To be impaired is to be different; valued attributes have been stripped away. Frequently, impaired individuals painfully discover that it is no longer possible to expect to be treated as a whole person. Those confined to wheelchairs often report, as one put it, that "people only see the chair, never me." The point is that an impairment, to varying degrees, imposes a social as well as a physical handicap and distance between ill persons and their significant others, complicating all aspects of life for the afflicted individuals.

Because of this, stigmatized individuals engage in various self-presentational tactics to minimize the impact of their stigma on others' reactions toward them. The most common one is to conceal their symptoms if their symptoms are invisible or easily disguised. In general, chronically ill persons are reluctant to disclose their illness to others and often experience stress from the fear of detection. On the other hand, some chronically ill persons purposefully reveal their stigma to others in order to downplay its consequences and convey the impression of having grace in the face of adversity. In fact, some of them take this a step further and try to turn their stigmatized condition from a liability to a benefit. At minimum, they point out that their experience with the stigma has made them stronger, increased their empathy for other stigmatized persons, or taught them to become better persons. In addition, some of them try to compensate for their stigma by becoming superachievers in other areas of their lives.

Occasionally, stigmatized people use self-deprecating humor about their difficulties to show they have come to terms with their disabilities (Jones et al. 1984). Sometimes people admit having a stigmatizing condition but argue that it is beyond their control and thus people should not form negative impressions because of it. Research, in fact, has shown that people seem to feel more justified in acting negatively toward those whose stigma is perceived as controllable than toward those whose stigma is not controllable, for instance, as seen in peoples' reaction to obesity (Farina, Holland, & Ring 1966; Rodin et al. 1989).

In a few instances, people seem to exploit their stigmatized condition for their benefit by advertising it, thereby eliciting sympathy, support, and other special treatment, and using it to excuse other problems. By playing up their handicaps, these individuals can blame their difficulties on their disabilities or on others' prejudicial treatment of them. I must confess I had thought that this would be the norm, that a lot of people would use this tactic, but I found it to be quite rare. What was even more uncommon was situations in which chronically ill people resigned themselves to the fact that others regarded them unfavorably and felt that nothing could be done either to counteract or to exploit their stigma. Only one respondent sadly stated, "I cannot do anything about what other people think of me, so . . . why bother worrying about what they think?"

For most respondents, the desires to maintain a positive evaluation of self and to continue prior relationships with others prompt them to engage in self-presentational tactics that counteract their stigma and to develop strategies for negotiating their positions. Despite all these efforts, however, chronically ill persons cannot avoid being stigmatized and discredited, and discrediting can occur during the course of encounters in which ill persons are subject to public mortification and embarrassment, often by surprise. Much discrediting, however, occurs in more subtle ways as when others simply assume that the ill person, because of certain limitations, is not capable of participating fully in decision making, even on his or her behalf, and is not given full adult status. For example, a couple of respondents mentioned the fact that health care professionals and family members make decisions concerning them without consultation. Indeed, people oftentimes talk about the ill person in the presence of that person as though she or he were not even there. That, in fact, seems to be a common occurrence, particularly for older people.

As awful as that sounds, Knudson-Cooper (1981) notes that those ill persons without significant others around them are perhaps even more vulnerable to new and more discrediting definitions as they become more and more disabled. Health professionals, especially physicians, become significant for these ill persons' developing definitions of self. I cannot support or refute that finding with my data, since with the exception of one person, all my respondents were living with their significant others. The respondent who was living alone at the time of the interview was living in the basement apartment of his sister's house, close to his significant other.

Whatever their social circumstances, since in most cases ill persons do not seem to be adequately informed about their conditions and the trajectory of their illnesses, they feel unacknowledged and unsupported, in short, discredited. Yet ill persons are afraid to share their feelings and fears with their caregivers, despite their interest in doing so. For instance, they feel that it is inappropriate to express emotional concerns to their doctors, both because they feel doctors are too busy for such conversation (Mitchell & Glicksman 1977) and because they believe the doctor will react negatively. They feel that they cannot afford to alienate the few people who still have an interest in their care. As one respondent, in discussing her anger at the doctor who "botched up" an operation, exclaimed, "Are you kidding? They hold your faith in their hands. If you cross them, they might not even try to do anything for you. And I want him to like me and try real hard!" Being silent, passive, and accepting is the perceived role of a "good patient" in general (Tagliacozzo & Mauksch 1979; Taylor 1979).

There are, unquestionably, areas of awkwardness and strain that develop when chronically ill people attempt to share their thoughts even with family members and friends. One of my respondents said that he hesitated about doing the interview with me because he did not want other "people to see [him] that way." Since I did not find him — or anyone — to have symptoms that frightened or repulsed me, I wondered how many others there were who would not grant an interview to a stranger because they thought that their symptoms were repulsive. Of course, my data are not representative of all chronically ill people; I interviewed only people who voluntarily agreed to talk to me. I probably missed the people who opted for total isolation because they believed themselves to be deformed and felt awkward.

Some chronically ill people become victims within their own families and among their friends because their disease raises such fear and anxiety among others that the patients are rejected, often avoided, and thus are unable to talk about the issues that are disturbing to them. In fact, Gordon and colleagues (1977) found that of the twenty problems most frequently mentioned by cancer patients, seven were of an interpersonal nature, such as difficulties in communication with friends about cancer, and in discussing the future with family, and the fact that people acted differently toward them after their diagnosis of cancer. The second most frequent problem cited in that research was lack of open communication with the family, which was mentioned as frequently as suffering physical discomfort (by 63 percent of the sample) and much more frequently than various problems with medications or overall treatment. Furthermore, if family members and friends perceive that the illness, symptoms, or treatments are stigmatizing, they urge or may demand that the ill person keep quiet about them, particularly if the symptoms undermine or involve loss of bodily functions. As Mitteness (1987) states, bodily control is considered a prerequisite to competent adult status, and lack of such control threatens to elicit judgments of personal incompetence.

Of course, the significance of the discrediting encounter depends on many factors, such as the situation in which discrediting takes place, the relative importance of the person(s) who discredit(s), the perceived extent of discrediting, and the amount of repetition of these discrediting events. The perceived extent of the discrediting can become very painful when the ill person either feels forced to accept the new definitions of self or feels that these definitions further erode an already shaky self-image. A respondent suffering from multiple sclerosis recalled the time she was sent to a rehabilitation center from the hospital: "Then they shipped me over to Passavant. And I was there for over three weeks because they didn't know, [were] trying to see if the nerves were going to come back, or they decided they weren't showing any signs of coming back, so they SHIPPED me out to rehab because they couldn't wait!" At the rehabilitation center, she was forced to confront and accept a reality for which she was not yet ready:

> Because most people that are in there are very depressed. They feel they're never going to be able to do anything again. So, their main motive [rehab staff's] is to get you motivated to do something, and at that time they were pushing me to type with my mouth because, you know, with a mouth stick because they didn't know if I was going to get the use of my hand back or not. And to use this apparatus they had for eating, but to me it was all [a] very grotesque type of thing . . . and, you know, I'm not going to—I don't want to do this! Because you're very negative to everything. And, of course, the people that are there are mostly, finally very handicapped, quadriplegic, parequads, aah . . . people that are in these wheelchairs.

Although the relative importance of those who discredit can shape the ill person's future and self-image, self-discreditation, on the other hand, is among the most damaging of the consequences of illness. It occurs first when the ill person can no longer adequately perform a function or express some previously valued attribute. It continues when the person defines that attribute or function as essential to a positive self-image. A respondent explained it this way:

> We're working on a job and a guy says we have to unload this off the truck. I have to say I can't lift it. I used to be very helpful before. I'm not helpful anymore like that. I have to think actually of myself now, and it bothers me sometimes because I wasn't that type of person. I was always helpful, wanting to give, you know. . . . That's difficult to have to say to people: I can't do that! I mean, my son—when we moved here and things like that—I really

couldn't really help because I don't want to strain my back and lay in bed or have to be in traction or something. So I have to limit myself. Well, it don't cause any difficulty, it just makes me feel that I'm not total, you know. Yeah, I'm not—A man is supposed to be macho, you know, and I'm not so macho because I'm sort of sitting on the sidelines. People are playing baseball, running around; you know, I can't take a chance sometimes. I always played baseball!

Hopper (1981) found that in patients with diabetes, self-esteem was rooted in their ability to be active and useful by their own definitions. She reported that these patients found their relations with those around them strained because of their illness.

In sum, most chronically ill people want to be treated as whole persons and known for attributes other than their illness. It hurts them to see how their illness clouds other peoples' judgments of them. As one respondent so perceptively stated, "People only see the chair, never me." Thus, chronically ill people expend much effort in self-presentational tactics and conceal their illness to counter and minimize the effects of their stigma. These efforts cause them additional stress.

3

Social Isolation: A Major Consequence

Lessened and impaired social contact and a sense of social isolation are among the more detrimental consequences of chronic illness. Social isolation refers to a negative state of aloneness or diminished participation in social relationships. Impaired social interaction relates to the state in which participation in social exchanges occurs but is dysfunctional or ineffective because of discomfort in social situations, unsuccessful social behaviors, or dysfunctional communication patterns.

Of course, the worse the illness (and/or its phases), then the more the probability exists that the ill persons will feel or become isolated. This isolation can happen in two ways: either the ill person, because of the symptoms, unexpected crises, difficult regimens, and loss of energy, withdraws from most social contact, or the ill person is avoided or even abandoned by friends and relatives. In either case, social relationships are disrupted or falter and break down (Strauss & Glaser 1975). All persons with long-term health problems are at high risk for social isolation. Social relationships are frequently disrupted and usually disintegrate under the stress of chronic illness and its management because chronic illnesses often involve disfigurement, limitations in mobility, the need for additional rest, loss of control of some body functions, and an inability to maintain steady employment. These factors tend to reduce a person's ability to develop and maintain a network of supportive relationships. As the illness takes up more and more of a person's time and energy, only the most loyal family members and friends persist in offering support.

Many factors may contribute or simply relate to the absence of satisfying personal relationships or lead to impaired social interactions. These factors include an altered physical appearance or emotional state, an altered state of wellness, self-concept disturbances, and inadequate personal resources caused by financial hardships. Social isolation probably occurs also because family and friends need to withdraw from the ill person to gain emotional distance and protect themselves from a painful situation, particularly if they are unable to help in alleviating the problems of the sufferer.

As they experience a restricted life, chronically ill persons become painfully aware that they cannot do many of the things they valued and enjoyed in the past. If they are able to participate on some level, that level is much diminished from that of the past. For instance, every chronically ill person interviewed named some cherished activity in which he or she could no longer participate. For some ill persons, the activity involves sports, for others, their work. These activities represent treasured social interactions with friends and acquaintances. As a respondent sadly noted, "I'd heard about people having kidney problems, but I never paid attention because I was always healthy, you know. So, I liked my job, I enjoyed working. I wish I was healthy, I could still work, because I met a lot of nice people and it was nice. And, you have to quit your job because of this!"

Some chronically ill persons interviewed regretted not being able to take vacations anymore, a change made not only for medical reasons but for a variety of other reasons. As one respondent put it, "I have to be on dialysis three times a week." Another one exclaimed, "I never know what can happen!" Financial considerations seem to be high on everybody's list. As a respondent explained, "I'm not working, so?". . . Another person said, "I'm only working part-time, and medications and stuff cost so much, we cannot afford it anymore". The financial burden that chronic illnesses so often place on individuals and families force some of these individuals to go to great lengths to keep working and to restrict all other activities in order to manage their jobs. A respondent who has to work every day no matter how he feels, stated:

> I just do what I have to do and that's it. I mean some days I'm feeling great and some days I'm not so great. . . . Now when I come home I just want to relax. I mean I just don't want to get up, get dressed, take a shower and go back out again. I just don't have the get up and go anymore. The energy, I want to save it. . . . I have to watch myself. It's a lot! People think, it's come on, we'll go out, we'll go running and we'll do this, we'll do that. I have to think twice. I'd rather just relax. Lay down and relax, you know. I don't know how you'd say, but I think more of myself now . . . than to go run some places just to be running, you know, is part of the problem. I can't do it!

As another example, a person afflicted with chronic renal failure requires the use of hemodialysis in order to survive. Such therapy often involves extensive time commitments on the machine and generally results in physical fatigue for many hours, sometimes days, afterwards. One's work responsibilities or schedule need to be rearranged; in fact, the work schedule needs to be very flexible. There are very few jobs that can accommodate such demands. Thus many persons undergoing hemodialysis are unable to maintain any type of employment or engage in social activities that other people take for granted. For instance, one such respondent stated:

> I just had a normal life. I just went to work and went home, spent some time with the family, went shopping. I still like to go shopping but . . . I miss that now. I can't walk very much; it's, you know, it bothers me. It's nice to be able to walk around. I can't take walks. Not just walks, but I used to walk to places – like to shopping. Instead of taking a bus or something, I used to walk. And I used to enjoy looking around in the shops, and now I can't. I miss that! I'm pretty much confined!

If chronically ill people cannot work, they frequently also leave their prior social worlds, alter their lifestyles, including changing their living quarters because of diminished financial resources. Either way, the result, in addition to the loss of a prior self-image, is social isolation, which also leads to emotional isolation. Indeed, most ill people experience daily reminders of their isolation, physical and emotional, as their lives become structured around and regulated by their treatments. Strauss and Glaser (1975), noted that some ill persons suffer not only from the intrusiveness of their treatments in their daily lives and from the related financial burdens, but also, from the knowledge that they are dependent upon their treatments or a machine to live (e.g., kidney dialysis, insulin injections). Thus they might begin to think of themselves as being less than fully human, and such thinking, together with a combination of physical incapacity and concrete restrictions, serves further to isolate them physically and psychologically from mainstream life and causes them to experience additional stress and frustration.

Part of the restricted life, in fact, is often caused by the harmful effects of the treatment itself. For instance, some patients find themselves to be as debilitated from their medications as they are from their diseases (e.g., chemotherapy for cancer patients can cause constant vomiting). Others view available treatments as devastating, sometimes more so than the disease itself (e.g., mastectomies). Part of the problem, as noted earlier, is that not all individuals are given adequate information and told about alternative treatments, and they have to rely on information from one practitioner or one perspective. These people often remain unaware of the available alternatives and of what else could be done to facilitate their attempts at adapting and normalizing their lives. As a result, the lives of many chronically ill persons are probably more restricted than need be.

As a matter of fact, since I interviewed more than one person suffering from a major illness, I soon realized that these individuals were not all receiving the same treatments for their illness, and when I asked if they were aware of a different treatment or a certain "miracle drug," they would either say no or tell me of instances when they approached their physicians with information they had gotten from other patients or from the media, only to be rebuffed by their doctors. For instance, an attractive 41-year-old black woman who had a mastectomy two years ago at a well-known hospital was not even informed of the possibility and given the option of immediate breast implant, a procedure that has been widely used in the last 15 to 20 years across the country. She subsequently found out about it from another patient and confronted her surgeon, to be told, "I didn't think it was important to you." Consequently, she had to go through the pain and expense of an additional surgical procedure to have the breast implant done. As she said, "I didn't want to give up my sex life."

Another major problem, as mentioned earlier, is inherent in the unpredictable course of many chronic illnesses. The uneven course of acute episodes of many chronic illnesses presents a threatening sense of uncertainty that prevents individuals from planning and engaging in social activities. This uncertainty and fear of acute episodes causes some patients voluntarily to restrict their lives, quit their jobs, limit their social engagements, and avoid many activities. Fagerhaugh and Strauss (1977) note that the greater the loss of control and the amount of potential embarrassment from the unpredictable nature of the illness, the more likely that person is to restrict life voluntarily. For example, a person afflicted with ulcerative colitis has to deal with the fear of emitting a fecal odor or encountering a bout of diarrhea at any given moment, resulting in embarrassment and/or humiliation, particularly during a sexual experience. The ultimate outcome is avoidance of future social and/or sexual encounters. One respondent told me that she does not eat a single thing for a couple of days before she has to attend a social and/or church function, so she can avoid any possible embarrassment. She told me that most of the time she simply does not participate, especially in any spontaneous activities, fearing potential embarrassment.

Social isolation is indeed a major consequence of a restricted life. Over time, the chronically ill have relatively few social contacts, even among family and friends. Since they no longer are able to participate in shared activities such as work, organizations, or shared leisure pursuits, such as games or sports, other people must come to them, which requires extra time and effort on their part. Hence, past reciprocity becomes altered and the chronically ill are left behind. Chronically ill persons frequently are unable to return support to others around them. Thus reciprocity, which is so important for healthy and balanced relationships, becomes impaired.

Furthermore, those who are chronically ill, unlike healthy people who can terminate relationships that fail to satisfy their needs, often are locked into unsatisfactory relationships because they fear losing or alienating those few who still care for them. Consequently, relationships of the chronically ill have less chance to be self-correcting and are more likely to contain conflict that generates ambivalence, dissonance, and, particularly, added stress. As one respondent, talking about a stressful relationship, nevertheless concluded, "I have to stick with her; who else would want me? Who else would put up with me, in my condition?" As mentioned, many ill persons voluntarily drift into social isolation because they do not have the time or energy to sustain their relationships adequately. Maintenance of friendships and relationships takes time and effort. Time is limited and priorities become reorganized because simply managing daily self-care takes longer when discomfort is high and energy is low. Time has to be taken for medical procedures and rest to restore energy, leaving very little time for social activities. Thus isolation seems to have a beneficial side as well, because it allows people to live at their own pace without distractions, thereby eliminating the pressures of social obligations and reducing stress.

However, for most people social isolation is experienced as a painful consequence of chronic illness because of the emotional deprivation factor. Therefore, many chronically ill people, especially older ones, welcome any social contact from whomever they can get it: door-to-door sales people, visiting nurses, meals-on-wheels drivers, and even interviewers. For instance, initially I worried that I would not find enough people to interview because I perceived that it would be a hardship or a nuisance for chronically ill people to talk to a stranger about their problems. I was wrong! Whatever their orientation or their illness, contacted people readily agreed to be interviewed simply because that seemed to be the only chance they had to talk to anyone at all about their problems. It seems that "nobody wants to listen," particularly those in the healthcare sector. "Doctors and nurses are too busy" and "Nobody wants to be bothered with my problems" are the kinds of feelings expressed by most people interviewed. In fact, some interviews lasted much longer, up to four to five hours instead of the anticipated two hours because the respondents were "so glad to have somebody listening" and paying attention to their problems. It seemed as though they did not want the interview to end. At the point of taking leave, several people actually said that they were glad that somebody cared enough to listen to them and invited the interviewer to "come back anytime!" — which in itself can be interpreted as additional proof of their social isolation.

Social isolation not only affects the individual, but the whole family as well, because management of a chronic illness usually reduces the whole family's free time and resources, leaving significantly less time and money for leisure activities. Coughlan and Humphrey (1982) documented that among the spouses of younger stroke patients, the loss of companionship and interference with social and leisure activities were described as the major reasons for a loss of enjoyment and quality of life.

Moreover, concern over other people's reactions causes other family members to withdraw from social functions. Many chronically ill respondents mentioned one way or another feeling guilty about the sacrifices friends and members of their families had to make, such as reducing their participation in social functions and/or giving up vacations. As one respondent mentioned:

> Well, my close friends, when we go out and stuff, they'll, you know, slow down just because I asked them to, or they see that I might be having, you know, a little bit harder time keeping up with them, like say, swimming or something. . . . I think it's real nice of them that they're doing that, and unless I'm having a real hard time breathing, you know, where they have to actually like, sit me and get me to calm down, I feel fine. But, if they have to do that, you know, sit me down or whatever, then I feel like I'm taking away some of their time. I feel like I'm being a little bit of a burden on them, because, you know, they have to go through all that, and I'm kinda like spoiling their fun and, you know, whatever they're doing.

There is bound to be ambivalence and resentment on the part of caregivers about the restrictions put on their own lives, and these reactions generate guilt in chronically ill people. Chronically ill persons' increased dependency upon close family and relatives may contribute to increasing conflict and hostility at home. For caregivers, the loss of the ill person as an active social partner and the demands of illness and treatment regimens, which reduce the time or energy available for social activities, may be important causes of problems and conflicts because they lead to social isolation for everybody involved. Respondents talked about the occasional comments made by family members and close friends to the effect that "this thing is taking over our whole life."

Furthermore, whether actual or perceived, episodes of being embarrassed, discounted, and otherwise devalued contribute to the social isolation of chronically ill persons even in their own families. When ill persons feel negatively identified, they begin to experience emotional isolation and remain unresponsive in the presence of others, which contributes to further difficulties in future periods of interaction. For instance, when asked if he discusses his health problems with other people, a respondent quickly and defensively replied, "Hell, no! Who wants to listen to my problems? I don't want to listen to yours. Who wants to listen to mine?" In short, "Other people don't want to be bothered with my problems" was a common sentiment expressed by many chronically ill persons interviewed.

There are also communication barriers in the social environment that make it especially difficult for chronically ill individuals to attain the support they need. For instance, many people seem to feel that it is desirable for chronically ill persons to remain as cheerful as possible. It is considered wrong for them to discuss problems they are having in coping with their illness or to focus on a negative prognosis. Those who discuss their problems are seen as coping poorly. One of my respondents put it this way: "I don't bore people with my problems! . . . Yes, I mean they'd rather not hear. . . . Listening to you complaining about something all of the time, you know, it ain't doing you any good, it ain't doing them any good."

Indeed, there is considerable evidence from the "death and dying" literature (Glaser & Strauss 1966, 1968; Kubler-Ross 1968; Pattison 1969, 1977) that people avoid seriously ill persons, discourage open communication with them, and give conflicting behavioral cues when in their presence. Many respondents mentioned getting a double message by those around them, messages telling them to ask for help if they need it, but meaning, in reality, "Don't ask!" Chronically ill people feel, as one respondent explained, that "people make empty gestures to make themselves feel better [and] they have no intention to help you. . . . They just want to look good, like they are nice people; . . . they are . . . but they just don't have time, whatever, so you get the message, don't ask! I don't rely on anybody, I take care of myself!"

In fact, people sometimes unwittingly perpetuate their own isolation. In other words, it is not clear how much of this lack of open communication is brought about by the chronically ill themselves and how much by others around them. An individual who might otherwise interact easily in social situations may fail to do so because of a visible trait related to a chronic illness, which thus leads to impaired social interactions. Even those persons with minimal visible dysfunctions or whose conditions are newly diagnosed are so anxious about the possible reactions of other people that the anxiety alone impairs their relationships. Many such people have concerns about disclosing their diagnoses, how and when to tell others, and what information to communicate. For instance, a young male respondent mentioned his difficulties in dating relationships; he stated that when questioned by potential girlfriends on why he walked with a slight limp, he would not tell them the whole truth about having a chronic illness that affected his leg muscles. Instead, he would just say that there was something wrong with his leg, implying a sports injury. In fact, he stated that he never "dreamed of being married" because of his problem. Thus he would not allow himself to get too close with any girlfriend and would "dump" girlfriends before "things got too serious" so he "wouldn't have to face telling them" about his situation. He further stated that it took him a full year before he told a girl he liked a lot about what was really wrong with him, because he expected her to dump him as soon as he told her. To his surprise and delight, she married him anyway.

The most common way ill persons drift into social isolation is in fact when they are removed from earlier social worlds by lengthy hospitalization and convalescence. Talking about her family concerns, a respondent explained:

I mean we had our ups and downs until '81; then I had a real severe fall, maybe when I fell down here in the house and I dislocated my arm, broke it, and I had severed – damaged – all the nerves to the point where I couldn't use this hand at all. So, there I was with no hand, and so I was already wearing a leg brace on the right leg and I had to keep the foot up. I was in the hospital for three months – which one month at a regular hospital, two months at rehab – and that was a little devastating, because that really put me back. I was, I finally just told them I had to get out of that hospital, I had people at home! I still had no use of either hand. . . . Still, I had to get home!

Indeed, unless their role in former social worlds is central to them, most chronically ill persons discover that each lengthy absence further weakens whatever ties they once had in that social world. People living alone and people of low socioeconomic status are more vulnerable to the effects of social isolation because they lack both the knowledge and the resources to gain access to social services. It is ironic that the more people need social services, the less they are apt to get them.

As the foregoing discussion indicates, chronic illnesses seem to foster greater dependence on others for self-care, self-definition, and value. At the same time, they tend to structure situations in which relationships become more strained and problematic. It is also ironic that even though the chronically ill may need and desire more intimate social contact to preserve their crumbling self-images and to monitor their images in their significant others' eyes, they themselves often become less capable of maintaining adequate relationships as they become consumed by illness. If they openly indulge in their suffering, guilt, anger, or other emotions, such as self-pity—emotions conventionally believed to be negative—they are likely to estrange further those who still take an interest in their care.

Part II

Managing Chronic Illness: Adaptation

If you haven't the strength to impose your own terms upon life, you must accept the terms it offers you.

—T. S. Eliot

The act of living itself is an adaptive process. By adulthood, everyone achieves a certain level of life adaptation, but chronic illness disrupts this achievement, because the additional burdens in dealing with the many problems of chronic illness diminish the capacity of individuals to respond in satisfactory ways.

Adaptation implies a balance between demands and expectations of a given situation and the capacities of an individual to respond to those demands. Failure to adapt, then, means that there is a discrepancy between demands and capabilities (Mechanic 1977). According to Dimond and Jones (1983), it is difficult to define and operationalize the concept of adaptation for several reasons. First of all, adaptation is dynamic; it changes as the environment changes. With respect to chronic illness, there are periods of progress and regress, depending on changes in the illness conditions, and chronically ill individuals must respond to those changes.

Adaptation is influenced by multiple factors and manifested in various forms. Individuals are not passive organisms; their responses to particular situations are conditioned by the success or failure of their past experiences, among other factors. Furthermore, adaptation takes place at an uneven pace within multiple spheres of life. Chronically ill individuals may be functioning well physically but be unable or unwilling to come to terms with the psychological aspects of dealing with life changes due to illness. Or they may be psychologically adjusted but unable to function as they see fit because of their physical handicaps.

Finally, adaptation is evaluated from many perspectives by different sets of criteria. Ill persons themselves, health care providers, family, friends, employers, and funding agencies (e.g., Workmen's Compensation) each have different sets of priorities and criteria for measuring different sets of role expectations. Consequently, as Dimond and Jones (1983) pointed out, there is considerable variation in an operational definition of adaptation, and this definition has changed over time.

For instance, some of the earliest literature in rehabilitation measured adaptation to illness only by focusing on very basic skills necessary for daily living, such as going to the toilet, dressing, eating, moving around within the living facility unassisted, and by considering basic communication skills (Katz et al. 1963). Although these skills are absolutely essential for achieving functional independence, the concept of adaptation has been broadened to include psychological and other social and behavioral aspects of life.

Psychological dimensions of adaptation are closely linked to social adjustment. Psychological concepts of denial, displacement, and projection (Christopherson & Gonda 1973; DeNour, Shaltiel, & Czaczkes 1968; Short & Wilson 1969); anger (Arnaud 1959); anxiety, frustration, and body image (Arnaud 1959; Buchanan & Abram 1975); and depression (Buchanan & Abram 1975) have all been used as indicators of psychological adaptation to chronic illness. Problem-solving skills, and learning abilities (Worden & Sobel 1978) as well as psychological well-being and life satisfaction, or "morale" (Carlson 1979; Dimond 1979, 1980; Holcomb & MacDonald 1973; MacElveen 1972; Simmons, Klein, & Simmons 1977), have also been used frequently as indicators of psychological adaptation. Furthermore, vocational activities, such as paid employment, changes in performance, and job disruption and/or satisfaction have also been used as primary indicators of adjustment (Carlson 1979; Garrity 1973a, 1973b; Goldberg 1974; Holcomb & Macdonald 1973; Hyman 1975; Morrow, Chiarello, & Derogatis 1978; Reif 1975; Smith 1979).

Most recently, participation in and enjoyment of family life, maintaining satisfactory relationships with friends and work colleagues, and leisure pursuits have been used as empirical indicators of social adaptation to chronic illness. Concern with these dimensions indicates an increasing awareness by health care professionals and researchers of the need to incorporate the concept of "quality of life" when measuring adaptation to chronic illness.

In fact, Strauss and colleagues (1975; 1984), in conceptualizing the relationship between chronic illness and the quality of life, identify a number of problems in adjusting to chronic illness. These include the following: the management of medical crises, the management of regimens, the control of symptoms, the reordering of time, the management of social isolation, the management of the disease course or trajectory, the processes of normalization, and the impact on family members. Without elaborating on the specifics of Strauss's discussion, the main point is that chronic illness makes great demands on the patient as well as the family and requires that an adjustment strategy be constructed, implemented, and worked at continually for adaptation to be accomplished. Indeed, demands on the chronically ill individual and/or family include developing and refining skills for daily monitoring and management of the health problem.

Management is no longer something that is done to a patient. That is, whereas patients who are acutely ill and immobilized for short periods of time are generally ready to subordinate themselves to the absolute authority of a physician who tells them what to do without explaining why, chronic, ambulatory persons who are ill but active over a long period of time are less willing to do so. Out of necessity, these mostly home-based persons do much of their own detection, diagnosis, and treatment. They also demand more information and a more active role in their own care, because they absolutely must in order to be able to function. For example, persons with chronic obstructive pulmonary illness have to learn to pace their activities so as not to overexert themselves, and they also have to learn how to use oxygen at prescribed levels during periods of shortness of breath.

Diabetic individuals have to learn to test their blood glucose levels, administer insulin, and adhere to a prescribed diet.

In fact, before they can do anything else, chronically ill people have to learn to accept the limitations of their conditions and learn to manage their own treatment and rehabilitation within the limits of their particular structural, social, and economic situations. Lorber (1967) points out that illness, like any other social situation, is a combination of physical reality and social evaluation and response. Hence, chronic illness often confronts afflicted people with the necessity for a change in lifestyle. These people, then, must also acquire the ability to strike a balance between either setting unrealistic goals for themselves that will inevitably lead to failure and surrendering all future plans and expectations of self, which will surely result in feelings of helplessness and hopelessness. Perry (1981), in his study of twenty patients diagnosed with chronic bronchitis and emphysema at two different rehabilitation facilities, found that when patients were encouraged to establish their own goals and priorities and try a variety of therapies to determine which one or which combination worked best for them, they reported a significant decrease in the number of symptoms.

In short, whatever their conditions or motivations, because of imposed disability, progressive deterioration, and the unpredictable nature of their illness, chronically ill persons have to adapt to changing conditions and make extensive adjustments in their lives. Major roles, such as wage earner and/or family caretaker, often must be modified. Accordingly, Feldman (1974, p. 290) defines adaptation to chronic illness as:

> coming to terms existentially with the reality of chronic illness as a state of being, discarding both false hope and destructive hopelessness, restructuring the environment in which one must now function. Most important, adaptation demands the reorganization and acceptance of the self so that there is meaning and purpose to living that transcends the limitations imposed by the illness.

It seems clear that this definition includes both behavioral and psychological dimensions of adaptation. It puts the whole burden of adaptation to chronic illness on the afflicted individual's ability to learn to live with the situation on a long-term basis and find purpose and quality in life within that context. Thus the definition also includes the concept of normalization.

Most of the definitions of adaptation, unfortunately, treat the concept of normalization as another adaptation strategy, giving it minor importance and thus creating a lot of confusion in the adaptation literature. In his definition, Feldman (1974) makes it clear that he is looking at two separate concepts, assigning normalization its due importance, yet he still seems to link adaptation and normalization together. I feel that these concepts are distinct from each other and need to be discussed separately. Thus this book shows the specific behavioral and cognitive strategies chronically ill people employ, as Feldman so eloquently put it, to "transcend the limitations imposed" by their illness.

First, however, I would like to clarify some of the confusion that might exist regarding the concepts of "adaptation" and "coping," concepts often used interchangeably in the health care literature as well as in everyday interactions between chronically ill persons and their caregivers. The next chapter attempts a clarification of these two concepts, and is followed by a chapter on adaptation. The process of normalization is examined in Part III.

4

Adaptation as Distinguished from Coping

Adaptation and coping are often treated as synonymous terms, but they are distinct from each other. Coping "is the special mobilization of effort and the drawing upon unused resources or potentials, [and] always involves some type of stress," whereas "adaptation is a broader concept that includes routine or automatized actions." Adaptation, in a psychological sense, "refers to *individual* survival, as well as to the capacity to sustain a high quality of life and to function effectively on a social level. In this use of the word, the focus is on outcome from an evaluative perspective — adaptive or maladaptive" (Cohen & Lazarus 1983, p. 611).

Initially, I also thought that "coping" and "adaptation" were synonymous concepts, that is, day-to-day symptom management strategies people employ to adjust to illness demands. It soon became obvious that they were indeed distinct from each other, although in many cases it is virtually impossible to make a distinction between these concepts because they are so interrelated. Indeed, while chronically ill individuals routinely deal with the daily demands of their illness, they are also trying to cope with sudden and/or unpredictable changes. As one of my respondents stated, "I can adjust to it [the illness], live with it on a day-to-day basis . . . but these damn changes, I can't cope with! As soon as I figure I can deal with this, manage ok, there is something else that I have to cope with." Adaptation, then, is what people have to do to function routinely, given the extra adjustments that they have to make because of their illness. Coping strategies are used when the regular daily routine is disrupted or no longer works because of changes either in the illness condition or the social environment.

According to Lazarus (1982), coping strategies function in two major ways. First, strategies are used to change the stressful situation for the better, either by changing one's own inappropriate behaviors or by changing the threatening environment. Second, strategies are used to manage the physiological or psychological outcomes of stress-related emotions themselves, so that they do not overwhelm individuals and damage their abilities to function or maintain morale. Lazarus calls this form of coping "palliative" because the goal is to relieve the impact of stress without actually altering the situation that caused the stress in the first place. Although he did not make a distinction between them, it is clear that Lazarus is talking about two different kinds of strategies: adaptation and normalization. What Lazarus calls palliative coping involves using cognitive strategies of normalization.

Thus, as I conceptualize it, adaptation strategies are instituted to take direct action implementing the necessary lifestyle modifications to adapt to illness conditions, together with behavioral normalization strategies to incorporate these changes successfully into a "normal" daily routine. If these efforts fail or the consequences of these combined strategies are less than satisfactory, then cognitive normalization strategies are used to deny or otherwise discount the importance of these changes, since not much else can be done, under the circumstances.

Of course, these strategies and coping styles all vary from person to person. Moos (1984) identifies three sets of determinants that account for an individual's cognitive appraisal of a serious physical disability and, ultimately, the coping strategies the individual uses to adapt to the illness. The three sets of determinants are, first, background and personal factors, which include age, gender, socioeconomic status, cognitive and emotional maturity levels, self-confidence, ego strength, philosophical or religious beliefs, and prior illness and coping experiences. Second, there are illness-related factors, which include the type and location of sympoms and whether they are painful, disfiguring, or in a body region vested with special importance, such as legs for an athlete or eyesight for an artist. Third, there are physical and social environmental factors, which include the physical living arrangements as well as family cohesiveness and support and social involvement and support.

Indeed, chronically ill persons are often in situations of potential threat or challenge that tax their ability to adapt effectively and carry out routine activities. At some time or another, all of them face events in their illnesses for which old and tried methods of handling problems are inadequate. Thus these individuals must learn how to cope with these events, adjust to new physical symptoms, and find ways to incorporate these changes into their daily routines so they can carry on as before. Moos (1984) further suggests that family and friends are also affected by the illness and will encounter many of the same or closely related adaptive tasks and use the same types of coping skills.

5

Factors Influencing Adaptation

Some adaptation strategies are mainly illness related and involve dealing with the incapacitation, discomfort, and symptoms of the illness itself. Depending on the specific illness, these strategies can involve controlling pain, dizziness, incontinence, extreme weakness, paralysis, the feeling of suffocation in respiratory ailments, and loss of control in convulsive disorders. Particularly, the course of illness, type of onset, kinds of limitations, and changes in physical appearance and functions interacting with situational variables affect the adaptive responses of individuals with chronic illness. These factors also influence the way people define the illness and attach meaning to it.

In other words, there are the challenges of the specific illness in question. Dimond and Jones (1983) point out at least three major characteristics of illness that are critical to the long-term adaptive responses of the chronically ill person. These characteristics are: the type of onset and expected course of the illness, the nature and extent of limitation, and the type and extent of changes in physical appearance and bodily functions. I will next discuss my data with respect to these three characteristics of illness; my study contributes the most to Dimond and Jones's first point.

First, the type of onset and expected course of the illness are critical factors in adaptation. Responses to chronic conditions that are acquired later in life involve the experience of adjusting to a loss of function, which is different from learning to live with a congenitally diminished or absent function, for the later does not involve the experience of loss. Chronic illnesses, because they involve losses or "little deaths," require adaptation on a daily basis (Burkhart & Nagai-Jacobson 1985). Sudden versus gradual onset of illness is a very important distinction. Gradual changes in bodily functions are easier to deal with than sudden, unexpected changes because gradual changes involve some sort of process of anticipatory socialization to the role of the chronically ill.

Dimond and Jones (1983) further state that the identified cause of illness is also a very important factor in adaptation to chronic illness. According to them, the way individuals respond, at least initially (e.g., with feelings of frustration, anger, or despair), is apt to be different depending on whether the chronic condition is the result of a genetic defect, pathology, accident, or some other cause.

My data reveal that in most cases chronically ill individuals are not informed about the identified cause of their illness, probably because there are no definitive answers. As discussed in chapter 3, my respondents *all* initially wondered, Why me? and came up with various speculations. My data also reveal that even if they had a pretty good idea about the cause of their illness, these respondents all reported experiencing feelings of sadness, frustration, anger, and despair at various times, no matter to what they attributed the cause of their illness. These same people also reported making efforts to overcome their negative feelings because they felt that these feelings were interfering with their efforts of learning to adapt to illness conditions.

Learning to live with a chronic illness is an ongoing task that demands skills beyond those needed for dealing with acute or self-limiting (e.g., disability) illness. With acute illnesses, disability is temporary, thus as soon as the crisis is over, afflicted persons can carry on and function as before. With conditions that result in permanent disability (e.g., polio, accidents, some surgeries), once people learn to adjust to their limitations and are able to incorporate them into their daily lives, they can carry on, certainly not at their previous level, but at least at a stable, though diminished, level of functioning.

On the other hand, because of the progressive deterioration and uncertainty inherent in chronic conditions, afflicted persons face threats to dignity and self-esteem, disruption of normal relationships, decreasing resources, and changes in lifestyle on a continued basis. As soon as these chronic sufferers can adapt themselves to one level of functioning, their circumstances change and they have to start all over again to learn to adjust to a new level of functioning. In some cases, there is a long period between changes in their illness trajectory; in other cases, the changes come rather fast. All these are problems for which no one can be completely prepared ahead of time. They may elicit a variety of responses, some of them self-destructive, including thought patterns that are self-deprecating and affective states such as anxiety, anger, and depression, at least at the early stages of illness, when these sufferers are the least prepared for what to expect.

Thus, the initial period following diagnosis of a chronic illness can be described as a period of disorganization and disruption in peoples' lives. Feelings of despair and hopelessness are often major hurdles that chronically ill persons and their families have to overcome. During this initial period, there are also cracks and separation within the support system of chronically ill persons, making their search for meaning in their misfortunes particularly difficult and painful. In many cases, it seems that the added stress of a chronic illness of a family member exacerbates an already dysfunctional family pattern, resulting in an increase of stress for all involved. As an example, a respondent explained that "my ex-husband, he couldn't understand why I cried all the time—you're nothing but a baby! And I couldn't make him understand the pain and there's nothing else I can do, and I figure if I cry I can release all that tension and at least feel a little better, so that's why I spent a lot of time in my room by myself, because I would just cry 'cause I wouldn't know what else to do with myself."

Indeed, what adds to the difficulties in dealing with the many problems of chronic illness is the fact that few people seem to be interested in personalized, prolonged contact with the chronically ill because the continual struggle to cope with day-to-day living soon becomes tedious, not only for ill persons and their families, but also for health care professionals, who are mostly cure oriented.

Even with no cure in sight, long-term and/or continuous care and support are required when dealing with the difficulties created by

chronic illness. Obtaining this support is particularly problematic
when patients are making the transition from acute care to rehabilitation or chronic status, because often the help and support that has been
available from health care professionals through a formal support
network is withdrawn before a new system of help and support is in
place. As one of my respondents so painfully found out:

> The arthritis specialist said there was nothing he could do, period!
> Not a thing he would recommend. . . . The orthopedic man— Well,
> it's strange, because this doctor is supposed to be very good, very
> busy. The last time my back went out I was at work and I came
> home and I called on a Monday or Tuesday—whatever, he didn't
> call me back. I called the next day, he is in with a patient. He'll
> call you back! He finally called me Sunday. . . . So, I lay in bed,
> of course, but I wanted some kind of reassuring or confidence from
> the doctor stating I'm doing the right thing, I'm not doing the right
> thing. He didn't call me. He finally called me and my wife was
> very upset about it!

In fact, people are routinely sent home from hospitals after their
acute crises have been controlled, under the often unfounded assumption that they will somehow know how to deal with their many
problems and somehow get the needed care. For instance, Mrs. X
was totally flabbergasted when her husband was being discharged from
a major area hospital after a series of extensive coronary bypass
operations with vague treatment recommendations and practically no
concern about his follow-up care. The two doctors present at the time
of the discharge—one the chief of surgery, the other a well-known
cardiologist—both seemed surprised at Mrs. X's suggestion about
hiring a nurse for a week or at least having a nurse-practitioner come
in a few times initially because she felt that her husband should not be
left alone for long periods of time during the day until he felt
physically stronger, psychologically more secure, and comfortable
with the treatment regimen. It apparently did not even occur to these
doctors to inquire about the social and psychological circumstances of
the patient, and they seemed to automatically assume that the wife
would take care of him. When it was pointed out to them that the
wife had a full teaching load and could not miss classes in the middle
of a semester, it did not seem to make a difference to these doctors.
The wife was still seen as responsible, and her concerns for her

husband's welfare were perceived as unwillingness to do her duty. She undoubtedly knew her husband and their circumstances better than the physicians and could predict potential problems. Nevertheless, the doctors did not agree that a nurse was needed; Mrs. X said that her husband felt "doctors know best," thus additional help was not utilized. Mr. X (age 54) was back in the hospital ten days later with major complications, needing additional surgery to save his life. Discharging chronically ill patients from hospitals without making sure that they have all the information they need and that adequate care will be available to them seems to be a common occurrence rather than an exception. Other respondents related similar incidents. Only the most assertive people seem to fare better; at least they demand to know what is being done for them. For example, a respondent stated, "I've gotten a world of information from every doctor I've ever been with because as I interrogated you at the beginning of this talk, I interrogate them. I am not bashful! I am not the kind that walks in, he takes my pulse and my blood pressure and then I walk out. I learned a lot from every one of them."

In addition, informal supports from family and friends change during this time, as the people who have provided the most help and support to a patient during the acute phase of the illness become "burned out" and in need of time to re-evaluate their help and support to the ill person. These peoples' lives have also been disrupted, and they feel a strong need to get on with their own lives, not only for personal and/or psychological reasons, but also for practical consider- ations. High medical costs, loss of income from the ill person, and uncertainty about future employment prospects not only affect the ill person but everyone in the family. Consequently, those connected to the ill person cannot afford to jeopardize their own jobs, and are caught in a dilemma. On the one hand, most would probably like to provide continuous help and support to the ill person, yet on the other hand, they simply are not able to do it for long periods of time without risking their own situations.

In contrast to the exciting aspects of sophisticated and mechanical technology directed at acute episodes, the rewards of treating chronic illness cannot be measured by cure but by the prevention of complica- tions and by helping ill persons function as best they can. These limitations make dealing with chronic illness a very tedious and never- ending project. Tedious or not, a lot of effort is directed by ill people and those around them at keeping the health problems controlled and in remission, while trying to control anxiety over the threat of full-blown incapacitation during exacerbations, so life can go on as normally as possible. But in the process, the effort is greatly taxing to personal relationships. Thus the primary adaptation strategies immediatly following diagnosis of a chronic illness involve finding practical solutions to control symptoms and learning to manage treatment procedures by establishing schedules to keep family disruption to a minimum.

Before they can do anything else, chronically ill people have to learn to deal with the incapacitation, discomfort, and symptoms of the illness and also learn to manage the special treatment procedures to control these symptoms. At the same time these people have to try to keep their feelings of despair and helplessness under control. But with notably few exceptions, once they leave the hospital, these people feel that they do not get much help from health care professionals on how to handle these tasks. Depending on the severity and unpredictability of the specific illness, these tasks can be overwhelming.

The process of learning to manage the special treatment procedures to control the impact of the illness can be described as a period of reorganization. Since physical symptoms disrupt and interfere with daily routines, they have to be managed and brought under control with medical procedures. Yet medical procedures and complex treatment regimens, which never completely eliminate the illness, also disrupt the usual patterns of living and place a drain on the time and energy of not only the chronically ill person but the entire family or support system.

In fact, the increasing sophistication of medical technology has created a number of ongoing tasks for chronically ill people. Chronic illness cannot be cured, but the effects of illness can be somewhat controlled with special treatment procedures. Since these treatment procedures also affect successful adaptation, certain strategies are needed for their management. These strategies are closely related to those dealing with illness symptoms, but they require the learning of new skills, which in itself can create some additional stress. For instance, diabetic patients have to be able to test their blood sugar levels and adjust their intake of food accordingly, and must learn the techniques of giving themselves the needed injections. One of my respondents described the long and complicated procedure of learning a system of caloric and sugar exchange so she could work out a diet to occasionally allow herself to eat the sweets she loves "without suffering the consequences." She also reported having to learn to adjust her insulin dosages not only to her food intake but also to her activity levels; she has taken up bicycling frequently because it helps her keep her blood sugar levels at a more even state. Similarly, long-term hemodialysis patients have to learn to monitor and regulate the machine themselves during lengthly treatment periods. Moreover, surgical procedures like mastectomy, colostomy, and tracheotomy; radiotherapy and chemotherapy with their concomitant side effects; and cumbersome braces all represent therapeutic procedures that create the need for additional adaptive strategies to be learned and implemented by chronically ill persons in their everyday lives.

Equally important, then, are strategies that consist of developing or mustering interpersonal communication skills to establish and maintain adequate relationships with health care professionals and other caregiving staff. These strategies entail learning to ask for additional information, medication, and services without appearing to be demanding (e.g., being labeled as difficult or a bad patient). They also entail learning not to express anger at the doctor or nurse when being ignored or when medical procedures go wrong or create additional problems (e.g., as in iatrogenic illness). Furthermore, these strategies include learning to deal with the disagreements among different physicians regarding appropriate procedures, and last but not least, they involve learning to handle the condescension, pity, or, as Ryan (1971) conceptualized, "blaming the victim" attitudes of some health care personnel.

Most of all, this whole process of needing to establish and maintain adequate relationships with caregiving professionals involves learning to be assertive enough to engage busy doctors and nurses in meaning-ful discussions on how a chronically ill person wishes to be treated as a whole person even though that person is incapacitated on some level, and physical improvement and progress is disappointingly slow. For instance, one of my respondents, a person who suffered from serious consequences of diabetes for more than ten years, recalled a particular incident that had happened to her some time ago, an incident that still seemed to make her very angry. She stated that not only was she not getting much help for her serious complications, but she discovered that she was being used as a "guinea pig" and as a teaching tool by a specialist without her consent, and made to pay for the privilege. She felt humiliated by the experience, and to add insult to injury, she was billed much more than usual for the longer office visit that this highly recommended specialist had apparently set up as a teaching session for his medical interns. She stated that she was not asked for her permission to be examined by those present, that she felt that she was being "harshly interrogated" about the "terrible condition of [her] foot" by people to whom she was not even introduced, and that her case was discussed in her presence as though she were not even present. This incident is unusual only because it happened to an upper-middle-class woman who later refused to pay the extra charges on her bill, assertively letting this physician know her reasons for it. She also found another doctor.

Unfortunately, many chronically ill people, particularly those with fewer resources, are subjected to these kinds of treatments, yet these people cannot afford to be assertive for fear of alienating those health care professionals who take some interest in their care. Furthermore, the frequent turnover and change in personnel, particularly among those who come into direct contact through patient care, makes this process of establishing and maintaining adequate relationships with these people an unusually complicated, stressful, and sometimes impossible set of tasks for chronically ill persons, especially for those with fewer resources. Many respondents talked about their irritations with health care professionals who seemed to be too busy, impersonal, and disinterested and who, in addition, seemed to make the patients themselves responsible for poor results, slow progress, or adverse consequences of prescribed medical procedures. Indeed, these are issues that plague chronically ill persons and cause them additional and unnecessary stress in their efforts of adaptation.

On the other hand, health care professionals are undoubtedly also frustrated with what they consider patients' noncompliance with prescribed medical treatments. What these professionals need to take into account is that physically painful procedures (e.g., injections), time-consuming regimens (e.g., dialysis), and treatments requiring major changes in diet, smoking and drinking habits, exercise, employment or climate change are perceived by ill persons on a cost-benefit dimension. Also, as noted earlier, people evaluate events in terms of previous life experiences, calculating the cost of making the expected lifestyle changes of the therapeutic regimen. These costs are weighed against the benefits of adhering to treatment.

Indeed, unless altogether helpless, as in the case of severe stroke victims, chronically ill adult persons are involved in managing and shaping their lives in the face of physiologic impairment and/or medical intervention. At the very least, these individuals have to work constantly at controlling their symptoms and implementing their treatment regimens. And since they can be perceived to be or actually are marginally beneficial, treatment regimens influence the adaptive responses to chronic illness. Some treatment regimens are simply unachievable given the social and/or financial circumstances of most people. Other regimens disrupt peoples' lives so completely or negatively affect self-esteem so greatly that people would rather opt to live with their symptoms than comply with the regimens.

For instance, hypertension is one of the most common chronic diseases in the United States, afflicting more than 60 million people. The incidence of the disease increases with age, and the prevalence rate among black Americans far exceeds that of the white population (Joint National Committee Report 1984). Hypertension is the major risk factor for coronary heart disease and stroke. Yet an estimated 40 to 50 percent of people with hypertension drop out of treatment programs within one year; of those remaining in treatment, the rate of compliance with the prescribed regimens is approximately 20 to 30 percent (Haynes et al. 1982). The primary reason given for the high attrition and low compliance rates is either the inability or lack of motivation of individuals to adapt effectively to lifestyle changes required by the prescribed regimen (such as dietary changes, weight reduction, exercise, smoking cessation, expensive medications, stress management, and regular follow-up clinical visits). Given the social and economic circumstances of most black people in our society, even suggesting and expecting them to follow such a regimen seems totally unrealistic.

In other words, what might appear to be noncompliance with prescribed medical treatments from the perspective of health-care professionals is actually in most cases rational and sensible behavior on the part of chronically ill persons, given their social and economic circumstances. People do not want to be sick, and they do not want continuous suffering. If it appears that they are not following prescribed medical regimens, it is either because these regimens are not helping them get better or the regimens are impossible to implement given their social circumstances. The type of onset and expected course of illness are critical to the long-term adaptive responses of the chronically ill because they determine the level of disruption in peoples' lives and relationships.

Second, according to Dimond and Jones (1983), the nature and extent of limitation is also a major factor in adaptation. It is difficult to describe these limitations objectively since for the most part they involve the perception of the sufferers themselves. Because illness is largely a subjective experience, persons with similar chronic illnesses who face some of the same disease patterns may have markedly different ways of adapting and, therefore, different outcomes to similar events. Consequently, behavior, the outward manifestation of adaptation, may be either adaptive or maladaptive, depending on the circumstances and the outcomes.

Obviously, there are differences in response patterns depending on the body system affected and the importance of that system to a person's occupation, lifestyle, and self-esteem (e.g., consider the loss of function in legs for an athlete or loss of speech for a professor). Sensory problems (vision, hearing, speech) require different adaptive responses than do problems associated with mobility. Furthermore, multiple impairments, relatively common among chronically ill persons are particularly problematic, sometimes requiring adaptive strategies that work well for one condition but are damaging to the other.

Finally, according to Dimond and Jones (1983), the type and extent of changes in physical appearance and bodily functions are also important factors in the adaptive responses of chronically ill persons, because they influence the extent to which persons engage in social or public activities (Melvin & Nagi 1970; Safilios-Rothschild 1970; Haber & Smith 1971; Moos 1977).

My data support Dimond's and Jones's assertions; in fact, most of the adaptations or adjustments made by chronically ill persons are behavioral and/or cognitive strategies used by these people to compensate for the nature and extent of their limitations and to cover up the type and extent of changes in physical appearance and bodily functions so they can continue to function at their premorbit levels. Since these adjustments are discussed in detail in chapter 6, I will now move on to other, related issues.

Most often, the adjustments chronically ill persons have to make take on the character of what Goffman calls compromised "role enactment," as individuals try to keep signs and symptoms at a level of side-involvement, in order to sustain their definition and participation in the situation for themselves and others on a somewhat permanent basis. That is, as Goffman (1963) noted, individuals usually try and are able to attend to bodily deviations within their situation set without the deviations becoming the dominant focus of attention within the situation. In fact, Goffman recognized that we are always faced with the biophysical fact of our existence, and that there will always be desire, in even the most circumspect of situations, to "shift slightly, scratch, yawn, cough, and engage in other side-involvements, affording creature release" (1963, p. 50); in other words, we try to contain within ourselves the deviations of our physical state.

Containment entails keeping our signs and symptoms at the level of a side involvement by suppressing them, not attending to them, concealing them, or shielding them, so that they may be integrated into the involvement contour and role demands and obligations of the situation. This activity becomes a major task for chronically ill individuals.

In fact, the more severe and the more visible the signs and symptoms, the harder the task of containment, and failure in this task may require abandonment of specific situational participation. For example, visible disfigurement (particularly that affecting the face), odors, sounds, and cumbersome equipment draw unwanted attention to afflicted individuals and often result in complete withdrawal from social interaction and obligations. For example, as soon as I arrived for the interview, one of my respondents said, "I was very leery about doing this interview because I don't want people to see me that way, if I can help it. At least, people I don't know." Another respondent stated: "I have to force myself. It takes me so long to get up for it and leave my house to come and meet my students. I can see the horrified looks, and even worse, the efforts made not to look at me when I am trying to speak. So, many times, I can't really make it!"

However, as Sarbin (1966) also noted, trying to keep signs and symptoms at the level of side involvement, most individuals engage in compromised role enactment rather than ask to be released from roles as suggested by Parsons's sick role concept, even though significant others may allow release from expectations of role obligations. Thus, the compromised role implies that individuals who are symptomatic modify, curtail, juggle, or negotiate their role enactment to remain involved in their situation set, in many cases throwing the definition of the situation into confusion. For example, the teacher just mentioned, as she became progressively more symptomatic, had to delegate more and more of her teaching duties to her students. As a result, some of these students became resentful and anxious, yet felt guilty for having these emotions.

Sometimes chronically ill persons make attempts to redefine the situation and try to modify the obligations and expectations of their roles to allow themselves to remain in a particular situation. They might do that because the situation is part of their identity and thus participation represents strong personal attachment (Goffman 1963). Indeed, the same respondent redefined the situation to indicate, "what better way to teach students than letting them get hands on experience, rather than just telling them what you want them to learn."

Citing several other researchers, Alonzo (1979, p. 401) perceptively pointed out that "situations may contain compromised involvement and role enactment to the extent that tolerance quotients (Lemert 1951), idiosyncrasy credits (Hollander 1958), and benefit of the doubt (Stone & Farberman 1970) are provided to an individual." These conceptions imply that there is a great deal of flexibility to a "normal definition of the situation," that is, they indicate how much dereliction in involvement a situation may contain before its definition is altered or collapsed. Alonzo (1979, p. 401) further noted that essentially "each individual is provided with a certain degree of idiosyncrasy credit, which he has accumulated by appropriate situational involvement and role enactment in the past." However, Alonzo notes that if no credit has accumulated or it has been exhausted, compromised role behavior will not be tolerated, and the individual may be asked to leave the situation or the situation may collapse if he does not take leave. For instance, the teacher mentioned was a well-liked, much respected individual with a lot of "idiosyncrasy credit" to her name, so she could remain in and modify the situation. Another individual in similar circumstances but with lower status and/or less credit would not have been tolerated. Another respondent, a well-established physician who himself had to be hooked up to a dialysis machine for several hours three times a week was provided with all sorts of amenities, such as private space and telephone, and even allowed to see some of his ambulatory patients during that time. In fact, the interview for this study was conducted during one of his dialysis sessions, at his request.

On the other hand, a young woman intern who developed a chronic, noninfectious, and, most of the time, nondebilitating condition, requested a more flexible working schedule so she could deal with her condition "if it flared up" and get the additional needed rest. She was denied this request because she was told that "it was against hospital policy for training interns." She was then forced to leave her position only a few months prior to her graduation, and thus could not complete her studies in her chosen specialty. As a consequence, she had to find a job at a less prestigious clinic working at the level of a paraprofessional.

Of course, this conceptualization points to the differential distribution of power in various situations. As Mechanic (1978) and Scheff (1966) both suggest, the status and power of an individual are important in attempting to define him or her as either physically or mentally ill. Indeed, some individuals with lower status and little power may be asked to leave situations when symptomatic, while more powerful individuals are able to use their own idiosyncrasy credit – or give the benefit of the doubt to less powerful symptomatic individuals. Thus, issues of containment and the success of adaptation must be evaluated while taking into account the relative status and power relations between the symptomatic individual and others in the situation.

As Alonzo (1979) so perceptively noted, situations vary in the degree to which containment and/or successful adaptation are possible, along many, sometimes interactive dimensions. For example, situations can be viewed as having bodily performance and impact expectancies. Performance expectancies indicate what physical or mental capacities, skills, reserves, or conditions are expected of participants in a particular situation. Impact expectancies refer to the consequences of bodily interaction with the situational environment (e.g., temperature, physical objects, dust, or strenuous situated activity). Indeed, each chronically ill person must assess whether, given his or her bodily, psychological, and social condition, he or she can adapt to the immediate demands of the situation and what might be the long-term consequences of participation.

As we can see, extensive adjustments, adaptation, and the condition that must be managed derive from signs and symptoms brought to or produced in the situation either as part of bodily background expectancies and/or from experience in some previous and similar situation. Thus on a day-to-day basis, afflicted persons must adapt to the sometimes variable manifestations of the illness process, and, of course, to the varying nature of situational participation. In fact, because of the variable trajectory of a chronic illness, situational adjustment is an ongoing and emergent process, because in contrast to Parsons's sick role formulation, chronically ill individuals feel that they must—or are encouraged and sometimes even coerced to—maintain normal activities and involvements, since their chronic condition is permanent. Thus the permanence and variable trajectory of chronic illness suggest that chronically ill persons, in addition to being responsible for continuing self-care, constructing effective adaptive strategies, and complying with medical regimens to control signs and symptoms, are also responsible for normalizing their situational participation.

In general, all this responsibility places an enormous burden for adaptation and normalization upon the chronically ill individual rather than upon the situation or lay others. Consequently, as previously noted, major roles such as wage earner or family caretaker often must be modified, sometimes with serious consequences to a person's identity and self-esteem, usually after a long period of suffering, when all sorts of possibilities have been exhausted as producing little success.

This later period of chronic illness can be described as the *resolution* stage in which losses are acknowledged, roles and expectations redefined, and the illness is incorporated in the life of chronically ill persons and their families.

However, since adaptation is a dynamic process, these periods of *disruption, reorganization,* and *resolution* frequently overlap and are re-experienced at various times as the illness progresses or new difficulties emerge. From the perspective of chronically ill persons, then, social adaptation is a series of never-ending challenges that must be met, since the most difficult factor in living with any chronic illness is its unpredictability. Indeed, the expected course of illness, particularly the element of uncertainty or unpredictability involved, seems to be crucial and in fact is the key element in the process of successful adaptation, because it determines the nature and extent of participation in social roles. For chronically ill adults, much of life centers around monitoring symptoms and maintaining regimens related to the illness, interrupted by occasional or sometimes frequent acute episodes. However, when symptoms are too intrusive and treatment regimens too demanding, they present problems that disrupt "normal" living, so various adaptation strategies are used to exert some control over these problems. These groups of adaptation strategies are generally implemented by all chronically ill persons, but their relative importance varies depending on the nature of the illness, the loss of function interacting with the importance of that function to a particular individual, the personality of that individual as shaped by past experiences and cultural variation, and the unique set of social and environmental circumstances. Particularly, the course of illness, type of onset, kinds of limitations, changes in physical appearance and functions interacting with situational variables affect the adaptive responses of individuals with chronic illness. These factors also influence the way people define the illness and attach meaning to it.

My research supports this extensive body of work, and shows that not all strategies employed by chronically ill people are intended to be strategies for learning to deal with illness symptoms and medical procedures. On the contrary, many strategies are used by chronically ill people to make themselves and those around them forget as much as possible about the reality of having to live with symptoms and medical treatments.

These particular adaptation strategies mostly involve normalization tasks, such as (1) preserving and maintaining a reasonable emotional balance, keeping anxiety and apprehension due to uncertainty in check, and fighting feelings of inadequacy and resentment; (2) dealing with the inevitable identity crisis by instituting the necessary changes in personal values and lifestyles; and last, (3) preserving relationships with family and friends, keeping communication lines open, in short, fighting social isolation. I conceptualize the particular strategies people use to deal with these tasks as "normalization efforts," discussed in Part III.

Part III

Living with Chronic Illness: Normalization

When life's terms offer you a lemon, make lemonade!

—Popular Folk Saying

Normalization refers to processes a chronically ill person uses to continue what that person perceives to be a normal life. There is a general presumption that people who work and participate in social activities lead normal lives; that is, they have the capacity to perform a variety of physical tasks, including self-care activities. Self-care is defined as the process by which persons deliberately act on their own behalf for the prevention of illness, health promotion, and the detection and treatment of health deviations (Levin, Katz, & Holst 1979). But with chronic illness, a person's capacity to perform these tasks becomes limited or activities become restricted as consequence of the illness.

Patient compliance, a concept related to self-care, is defined as the extent to which a patient's behavior coincides with the prescribed treatment recommendations (Sackett & Snow 1979). Studies that examine patient compliance in chronic illness find that adherence does

not necessarily result in achieving desired treatment goals, nor is it
directly related to control of the illness and/or symptoms.

There is no effective way for measuring patient compliance, in any
case; these studies largely rely on patients' self-reports, and since there
are cultural norms against noncompliance with medical advice (e.g.,
people say the doctor knows best), there is a strong possibility of bias
toward the socially acceptable answers given by patients. We really
cannot know if chronically ill people are adhering to treatment
regimens or deviating from them without admitting to it, because they
may be afraid of being blamed by their caregivers if something goes
wrong.

In any case, as noted in the previous chapter, often ill people are
held responsible for poor results, slow progress, or adverse
consequences to treatments even if they follow the prescribed
treatments, perhaps to avoid an alternate and logical explanation that
the treatments themselves are not effective. For instance, one respondent recalled that at the very beginning of her illness her doctor was
very hard on her, yelling at her when her blood sugar levels were off
because he did not believe that she was complying with her diet
restrictions, although she told him that she was. He then had her
admitted to the hospital to control her dietary intake, but her blood
sugar levels were still way off, as is the case with many diabetics until
the right formula is found through trial and error. Yet the respondent
reported to me that her doctor continued to blame her and in fact had
her transferred for a few days to the psychiatric ward of the hospital
for evaluation because he felt that she had "personal problems" that
kept her from complying with the treatment regimen. The respondent
insisted that at the time she was strictly following her doctor's orders
because she "didn't know any better and was too scared not to follow
them, anyway." Yet, as she recalled, she was still blamed by her
doctor for noncompliance.

In contrast, a couple of respondents openly stated that they deviated
from the prescribed treatment recommendations quite often, but would
not even dream of telling their doctors about it. For instance, the
respondent who was using "horse medicine" for his arthritis did not
think that his doctor would appreciate it or approve of it. Another
respondent reported changing her medication herself "because I
thought it was better for me. I don't know, I just didn't like the fact
that I always had to go to the doctor and spend money for the

examination and you know, do other stuff, when I could just go to the store, and the contents of what he was running me a prescription for were pretty much the exact same contents that were in the Primatine, so I just switched, then."

Other chronically ill persons stated that they tried telling their doctors about deviating from the prescribed regimens because of certain problems they were experiencing and/or because some of these regimens were difficult to implement or downright unfeasible. These people reported not being listened to or being scolded for noncompliance. So people may do what they feel they have to without reporting deviations to their doctors. The 23-year-old asthmathic woman respondent just quoted elaborated on why she does most of her own "doctoring":

He's [her doctor] still a fairly good friend that I've known for a long time, but as far as trusting his diagnosis, I have little, I kinda sit back and look at it a little closer before I—Because everytime something happens, it turns out the doctor isn't right. He has to go through a whole series, and he might bark, saying wait. Well, let's face it, I know what's going on inside me or whatever. You know, it just takes him a long way to go about it medically, than the same thing I've been telling him, but of course, being the doctor, he has to do it the scientific way. I don't, I think it's this, and he has to go through all the tests and say, Okay, you were right, but it took me longer to figure it out.

In order for treatment to be effective, information in the doctor-patient relationship must flow in both directions. In fact, Julius Roth (1963) documented his experiences as a patient in a tuberculosis hospital by writing Timetables a book in which he provided not only insight into the illness experience but also valuable insight into the means and reasons by which doctors limit or control the amount of information shared with patients. Since patients, especially chronically ill patients, are normally not aware of their prognosis or the results of laboratory tests and X-rays unless their doctor decides to inform them, they deviate from the prescribed treatments if they think that these treatments are excessive. Roth (1963) also noted that on occasion doctors and nurses will even deliberately limit communication with patients if it interferes with their work or might lead to patients' discovering their mistakes and shortcomings. Whatever the reasons, health care professionals seem to give relatively little time to providing medical information and answering questions, and they spend virtually no time in finding information about patients' circumstances, at least to their patients' satisfaction. Waitzkin (1976) reported that one minute of a 20-minute appointment was given to exchanging information with patients.

As we can see, there are real limitations in applying the concept of patient compliance to effective management of chronic illness. Since treatment of chronic illness is usually on an ambulatory basis, primary responsibility for the daily management of health problems rests on the chronically ill persons themselves.

Furthermore, since persons with chronic illness generally continue their usual social roles and responsibilities, they cannot assume the sick role. Thus they need to incorporate the appropriate health or illness behaviors into the context of their daily lives, in other words, to live with their limitations. As one of my respondents, a man who works in the construction trade and gets paid only for the actual days he works, stated:

> I have to work every day. I have no choice in the matter, and I live with the pain. I mean, it takes me awhile in the morning 'til I get up to [be] normal, you know! . . . Well, in the mornings when I get up, I can't stand straight; it takes time for me to straighten myself up, you know. When I wash to get dressed in the morning, I'm sort of stooped over and have to do exercises and try to keep it limbering, it flexible as possible. I mean it will never get the way it should be. . . . A therapist, and she taught me how to live with what I had by doing certain exercises—how to sit, how to stand, you know! And when I drive I put something behind my back, keep it arched, and I've been living with it. We don't get paid when we are sick. We don't have sick leave or anything like that, so when I'm off, I don't get paid, so it's hard on me. And the union would pay, but they pay after seven days for sickness. I mean it bothers me every day, . . . so I just cope with the pains, I guess, and whatever, and do whatever I have to do!

A highly paid executive expressed similar concerns:

> I didn't have any choice, being responsible for and raising and feeding and educating seven children, I had no choice. I had to just

go on doing what I had been doing because I had to earn the money to pay the mortgage, to pay for the land, insurance . . . what can I say? I had no choice. So . . . not by any great strength of my character, maybe by, of course, circumstance, I had to accept it and work around it. . . . Cutting back on working from 80 hours a week to probably 60 or 55. What else could I do?

Another respondent, a wife and mother, explaining her reactions to finding out that she had a seriously debilitating illness, stated her reasons for going on with her life and continuing to take care of her responsibilities despite her illness:

Well, I was very upset, because I had these four little kids and my husband and I were very active people. And, oh Boy! You know, we were very sporty, and we liked to go out with sports and dancing. And we were not the intellectual type, we were more like, . . . Let's get up and go do things! It was very hard! Although I was still able to do things, get around, you know. Just that if I got too tired, then the leg would give me problems. So, I just sort of kept going, you know; you have got four little kids, you know, you don't stop.

In sum, self-care not only emphasizes activities to manage illness-related problems but also encompasses a whole range of related behaviors that are essential to overall well-being. A lot of self-care behaviors as well as behaviors that appear to be noncompliant with medical advice are essentially rational normalization strategies from the perspective of chronically ill persons.

Normalization refers to attempts of chronically ill persons to establish, maintain, or pretend to be living as normal an existence as possible, despite their illness symptoms, handicaps, and complicated treatment regimens. In fact, chronically ill persons expend great effort to try to convey to others the impression that their lives do not significantly differ from that of normal or so-called healthy people. In other words, more than average people, they seem to engage in impression management. They may try to convince themselves as well. Darling and Darling (1982) noted that the most common management strategy in dealing with chronic illness is normalization. Normalization, however, is more than a strategy; it is a complicated process that has both behavioral and cognitive components involving many strategies (Birenbaum 1970, 1971; Darling & Darling 1982; Roskies 1972; Vosey 1972).

The concept of normalization itself must be further examined and clarified. Knafl and Deatrick (1984) state that the term "normalization" appears quite often in the literature on how families respond when one of their members has a chronic illness or disability and reflects an underlying assumption that all families should be encouraged and helped to attain a normalized existence. These researchers rightly point out, however, that "definitions and applications of the concept vary considerably across investigators" and that it is therefore important to distinguish "among the various ways families manage chronic illness and disability" (p. 2).

Normalization strategies are not inherently adaptive or maladaptive. They may be appropriate for one person or one situation, and not another. Furthermore, strategies that may be beneficial in some circumstances may become harmful if relied upon exclusively. As a general observation, the most successful normalizers I interviewed seemed to be people who were, by their own admission, flexible, and willing to take chances on their own and experiment with various, sometimes nontraditional, procedures. For example, one of the respondents mentioned earlier stated that he had tried virtually every traditional remedy prescribed for arthritis with no discernible beneficial results; then he turned to: "horse medicine! . . . So, I ended up, somebody told me that there was a solvent strictly for horses — got label on the bottle; you cannot buy it in the store. You . . . order it. I have been rubbing my knee. . . . I found out from somebody, but it was no doctor. You gotta get a release. So, I got my release! . . . (laughing) I don't think I ever told him [his doctor]."

My data reveal that newly diagnosed people seem to be more cautious than long-term sufferers about experimenting on their own, saying that they are strictly compliant with prescribed treatments and are less willing to try various new procedures. Aside from the possibility that some of these respondents are giving the socially desirable answer, I speculate that these persons are also either unaware of — or are denying — the severity and unpredictability of their illness. A strong possibility might also exist that since these people are at the beginning of their illness trajectory, they have not been through as many setbacks and disappointments as long-term sufferers. Consequently, these newly diagnosed people are more optimistic and hopeful about the availability of effective medical treatments. Believing that these treatments will work; they are more compliant with the prescribed regimens than long-term sufferers.

Conversely, long-term sufferers seem to be more inclined to try new procedures and experiment, or at least say that they are, than those diagnosed in the recent past. They seem to project, as one respondent put it, a "what is there to lose" attitude; thus they will exhaust all possibilities. As a respondent explained:

> I went to a chiropractor first. I've tried a naprapath. So, I've not went to one man, I mean I've went to these other people, and they've done . . . not terrific. They didn't do anything that was worthwhile, so I went—my main doctor said, Call the orthopedic man. I said, OK! It [his back] went out on me on a Sunday. Monday I went to a chiropractor, Tuesday I went to a chiropractor, still the same thing. Finally, I went Wednesday to the orthopedic man. He examined me, he says, Your back is out!

Some long-term sufferers say that they are willing to try all sorts of things suggested to them by their doctors, friends, and relatives. Yet, at the same time, these individuals feel, as one put it, "It probably will not work, but I'll try it anyway." They assume a wait-and-see stance, going through the motions. On the one hand, these people might be making realistic assessments of the costs and benefits of a particular treatment, and thus using adaptation strategies. But on the other hand, they may need to try different things in the hope that one of them will work (as one respondent said, "You'll never know, it's better than doing nothing") without really believing this, thereby protecting themselves against potential failure. The 50-year-old construction worker quoted earlier said that he does take his prescribed medication regularly, even though he does not think that it does him "a lot of good. I just take it. I figure the worst it could do is not help me at all. O.K! . . . It's sort of like a crutch."

A few long-term sufferers, however, stated that they will not even attempt to try different regimens, even though they know about them. In fact, a few respondents told me of various available "cures" that they had not tried because they did not believe these cures would work for them. Some of them were discouraged by their doctors in their attempts to try different treatments. Even the more adventurous patients seemed to get intimidated by their doctors about experimenting with nontraditional remedies. For instance, the 50-year-old male respondent just quoted was so desperate at one time that he even went to an arthritis conference for medical people to find out about "new cures . . . some other kinds of shots used in other countries . . . in Mexico," and informed his doctor about them, and asked him: "What about me? What about shots for me? All these other people are getting these other shots for backs. . . and so. . . . He just said, It won't help. I didn't want to push the issue, you know. Well, if it won't help, it won't help!"

In fact, my data show that chronically ill persons, whatever their approach, seem to learn to deal with their problems by trial and error mostly because they have to. In general, these people are on their own either because there is not enough information on how to deal with specific difficulties created by the illness and/or available treatment procedures, or they are not given all the needed and available information by their health care providers.

With the exception of a couple of people, my respondents talked about their frustrations with not getting much information from their doctors about their illness, its prognosis, and available treatments or alternatives. For instance, a respondent who is a nurse indicated that she learned a lot more about her illness from patients in the hospital or high school friends' parents. "I ask them questions about how things went and what medication they're on, particularly people who are postsurgical. I know somebody had surgery for it, I held a whole discussion on how it was. I may be totally different from them, but out of curiosity and partly I feel comfortable asking things like that 'cause I'm a nurse . . . but partly out of curiosity for myself. . . . What it was like . . . or what the surgery was like. How long it was from the time they first were having symptoms till they had to have surgery? . . . It would give me some idea of what the future holds."

In fact, most of my respondents indicated that upon diagnosis, they learned more about their illness and the available treatment procedures from friends, particularly friends who are nurses; from other chronically ill people; and from the media, rather than from health care professionals in general, particularly their physicians and nurses they have come in contact with in hospitals. As one respondent stated, "once they told me, I started, you know, I went in the encyclopedia and I was reading up on it to see what exactly it was that I was supposed to be going through." Even the two interviewees who stated that they were satisfied with the honest and forthcoming manner of their doctors admitted learning about their illness mostly from books and magazine articles. Their appreciation was for their doctors' help at least providing them with the appropriate references for locating the needed information.

On the surface, it might appear that all these long-term chronically ill persons, those who are pessimistic experimenters as well as those who seem to have given up altogether, are not adjusting well to their illness conditions, or in Parsonian terms, are not trying hard enough to get well. In reality, these persons eventually discover that some of the advocated cures are not feasible because they are either too costly or too disruptive to the whole family situation. Furthermore, many of these sufferers have been disappointed before by "magical cures," and thus they are simply being cautious. They are all using normalization stategies to avoid potential failures and thus to protect their self-esteem. They are also trying to live as normally as they can in spite of their illness. As Kinchloe (1986) indicates, chronically ill persons have a need for meaningful and satisfying activities that can be undertaken despite the presence of illness, yet they encounter many difficulties in their efforts to normalize their lives.

6

Factors Affecting Normalization

A primary set of normalization tasks involves preserving a reasonable emotional balance by controlling upsetting and negative feelings aroused by the illness. Anxiety and apprehension caused by not knowing what will happen next, feelings of inadequacy, and resentments in the face of difficult demands are understandable and inevitable, yet these feelings must be managed so that the more mundane tasks of learning to deal with these demands can be undertaken.

Many respondents talked about having to control negative emotions such as a sense of failure or inferiority, and two people in particular talked about feelings of self-blame, possibly for past wrongdoings. Two other persons mentioned being extremely depressed, even suicidal, particularly at the onset of their illness:

Well, when I first come out of the hospital, the first four months, I was, like, depressed. Like I told you, I had that terrible pain in the arm. . . . I thought I don't want to go on like this, you know, . . . so I thought of committing suicide. . . . Why go on living like this, you know, but just in agony and going to dialysis three times a week. But I got used to going to dialysis and my hand stopped hurting. Still, I'd like to change things so I could – but my main thing – It's ok!

Another respondent expressed similar feelings upon finding out her diagnosis:

Oh, God! I felt like they had condemned me to the wheelchair. It was my biggest problem, point blank: that you are going to be a cripple, you just have a few years to go before you're in that wheelchair! You won't be able to do nothing for yourself! And, that first night when I was lying in the hospital, I just thought, you know: I don't want to be like that, I don't want to be in a wheelchair, I don't want people waiting on me. I'd rather be dead, and that's exactly what I thought. I thought, if this thing gets much worse, I'll just take all them pain pills and I'll just sleep. That's terrible, suicidal! You never know if people will do it or not, and when I hear these people say, Oh, I could never do nothing like that or I could never talk like that; they don't know what they can do. . . . I find myself, probably psychologically, forgetting to take the medication, and it's crazy, I paid for it. Again, but at the time you want to feel once again normal, you know. That's the only way I can put it, because you aren't normal when you're dealing with all of those things, everyday. I don't know, I think I've worked myself now when I find myself getting really uptight, I can just sorta calm myself down and say, Hey, it's not worth it, you're not gonna get – Nothing is worth that. Everything is gonna turn out the way it's meant to be anyway, so why worry about it, why get upset about it? Just let it go! . . . I try not to give in to it like I did. When you give in to it, it's gonna get you!

As the examples indicate, most of these people eventually learn to manage these emotions, especially when the initial acute episode of the illness is brought under control and they begin to adjust, more or less, to their symptoms and start mastering their treatment regimens.

A related set of normalization tasks consists of preserving a satisfactory self-image and maintaining a sense of competence and mastery despite all the undesirable changes brought about by chronic illness. Changes in appearance and body image as well as difficulties in physical functioning threaten to create an identity crisis. For example, chronically ill persons who must rely on mechanical devices like wheelchairs to get around or on hemodialysis or pacemakers to sustain their lives have the task of coming to terms with, as one said, a "half-person, half-machine" body image. A dialysis patient exclaimed: "This damn thing [pointing at the hemodialysis machine] runs my life!" These and other changes, such as physical deformities, unsightly scars, or permanent weakness, must be incorporated into a revised self-image, and they often necessitate a change in personal values and lifestyle. For example, one of my respondents who had high aspirations and according to him, "a good chance of becoming a college football star" had to settle for "helping kids to develop their talents in sports, and coaching a women's softball team . . . at a local Park District." Thus this set of normalization tasks involves realistically defining the limits of disability or competence and readjusting goals and expectations according to changes brought about by illness conditions, so afflicted people can more or less function in their usual social roles.

However, even if they are able to, resuming self-care activities and performing customary social roles are particularly difficult for chronically ill people after a long period of enforced passivity during acute episodes of the illness trajectory, as, for example, when these people are confined to hospital care. On the other hand, family, friends and health care professionals very often assume that chronically ill people are ready to resume their usual activities once the acute episode of their illness is brought under control and they are sent home from the hospital. In reality, many chronically ill persons are physically and/or psychologically not able to fulfill the expectations of those around them, at least not initially, because of illness-imposed dependence. Yet these people are often pushed into resuming their social roles and obligations much sooner than they are able to, and accused by those around them of malingering if their performance is less than adequate. Some chronically ill people report being told, as one of my respondents said, "You'll feel better if you do things, get out more." Another person stated that she is constantly told to "keep busy, to get your mind off your illness."

Other chronically ill individuals seem to have the opposite problem. Those who feel capable and willing to resume their former social roles and obligations as soon as possible are kept from doing so by the overprotectiveness of family and friends. These people report being told, as one of the respondents explained, "You've got to take it easy, you're doing too much." Another respondent reported being constantly made aware that "you are not ready yet; remember, you're sick."

Thus far, research on the influence of family relationships has yielded apparently contradictory findings. For example, there is research indicating that supportive family relationships are very important (Klein, Dean, & Bogdonoff 1967; Hyman 1972; O'Brien 1980). On the other hand, some research shows that supportive families can increase dependency and thus hinder successful rehabilitation (Hyman 1971). There is also research describing the changing scene of family dynamics at different stages in the course of illness (Klein, Dean, & Bogdonoff 1967; O'Brien 1980; Croog & Fitzgerald 1978) and the enormous stress that chronic illness places on family relationships. All these findings are valid and not necessarily contradictory. Furthermore, they help us understand the dilemma chronically ill persons find themselves in during their attempts at normalization.

Cockerham (1981) points out that the relationship of family to effective adjustment to living with a chronic illness is not a simple structural matter, but rather must be understood in its qualitative dimensions. Thus, the strength or weakness of the bond in relationships may be the crucial factor in the process of successful normalization, not simply the presence of another—spouse, parent, or other relation. For example, a respondent talked about her relationships in the following way:

> Sometimes I feel slightly sorry for myself that I can't do all the things that everybody else can do. . . . I think of myself as probably not quite as a fun mother, that I can't do as many physical things . . . or a fun wife; I wish I could dance around more and all that. . . . My husband doesn't get into real strenuous activities and I think there is, I know there is, a certain amount of uncertainty in his mind about what's bothering me. . . related to it, so I think that he's unsure about when to keep at home and what would happen to me. It's not like he goes on hoping. . . . In fact, we never really talked about how he feels about it. He'll ask me sometimes if I'm alright. He says I'm falling behind walking or whatever.

Another respondent stated that:

> It's probably one of the reasons my marriage failed. I—you always
> need somebody, but I always felt like the wrong one in the
> marriage. I always felt that I was wrong and I didn't have anybody
> to tell what I was going through. The relationship just sort of
> deteriorated because—Well, that's when I finally called off the
> marriage, because I couldn't deal with that problem and my pain
> too. I just couldn't deal with the both of them. It was bringing too
> much . . . to my life, and it was after we got separated that I
> started thinking about me.

Indeed, people with poor or deteriorating family relationships may add
to the problems of adjustment in their process of normalization by
trying to please or accommodate those around them.

In either case, whether because of the need to depend on others for
self-care activities and emotional support or the need to evade
overprotection, chronically ill people find themselves in distressing no
win situations. Yet, most of them try very hard to find a personally
and socially acceptable balance between accepting help when they need
it and taking an active part in determining the direction and quality of
their own lives. As one respondent remarked: "as long as they don't
say, Oh! Well, you can't do that because you have asthma, you
know. Let me be the one to decide if I can or can't do that. . . . I
know my own restrictions." In short, one of the hardest tasks for
chronically ill people is to convince those around them that they
themselves should be the best judge of what they can or cannot do and
of what is best for them. Furthermore, they have to do it without
alienating those persons who still care for them.

A last set of normalization tasks includes fighting alienation and
stigma to prevent social isolation. Preserving relationships with family
and friends while experiencing a sense of alienation caused by the new
identity as a patient or, worse, as a dying person or, at the very least,
as someone who is different from others makes this set of tasks very
stressful and difficult for chronically ill people. As one of my respondents painfully stated:

> I have a step-daughter. . . . I haven't seen her for over three
> months and she—well, she has two children. One is 2 years old,
> and I sort of feel bad that I don't get to see them more often. . . .

But before I got sick, this was funny, we used to see each other a lot. We used to visit a lot! She had me over to her house, I'd have her over here, and then we used to go places. And, you know, we'd take her little daughter, S., to the amusement parks – that's when I could walk, you know. And we used to go to Wisconsin. We used to – to be close! We used to see each other a lot! Call each other up every week and everything, and now she doesn't have a phone because she can't afford to have a phone. She wrote me one letter in the past three and a half months, and I wrote her one letter, and that's it. I mean – I mean I feel kind of bad about that. We were very close. We were also going and doing something with the kids and her husband and my son and that, we'd get together, and now it all just stopped! . . . My two sister-in-laws, I used to see them once in a while. I haven't seen them . . . in a while now. I guess when you can't do things, they sort of stay away from you.

This sense of alienation, starting with the physical separation occasioned by an initial hospitalization, is often enough reason to disrupt normal relationships with family and friends. Indeed, serious long-term illness makes it extremely difficult to keep communication lines open at the very time when emotional support and comfort are most essential.

Many factors affect whether one can achieve normalization, factors such as the severity and visibility of the symptoms, their unpredictability, the difficulties of special regimens, divergent perceptions of disability between ill persons and their care givers, and last but not least, the availability of resources, both monetary and personal. According to my data, the first three factors, particularly severity and visibility of the symptoms, seem to be the most crucial factors in achieving or hindering normalization; most of the normalization strategies employed by my respondents are intended to counteract the consequences of these factors.

Of course, some symptoms are not visible, others are misread or perceived incorrectly, and certain symptoms are more likely adversely to affect interaction than others. As a young diabetic woman, discussing the differential treatment she received throughout her school years, recognized:

In kindergarten, I started this whole thing. And then when I went into first grade, first through eighth in grammar school . . . I had my two-snack rule. One in the morning and one in the afternoon. I had to eat in class when it was definitely forbidden in the parochial school. . . . I was the first one in the school – oh there was one other girl. . . . I wasn't the only one, but it was always explained to each child; There is this to deal with in this person's life, respect it! And, I never, I can sincerely say, I never had anybody come to me and say how terrible, or to laugh at me, and I think one of the reasons is because it wasn't actually a physical deformity.

When symptoms are invisible or other people are unaware of the illness, chronically ill people have the option of "passing," that is, of engaging in normal interactions. The fact that most people I interviewed said that they did not tell others about their illness unless they absolutely had to might be an indication of "passing." In fact, controlling information or covering up is the major normalization strategy used by these people to keep themselves from being stigmatized.

Covering up allows chronically ill people to view themselves as they would prefer to be viewed by others. It includes keeping the signs and symptoms of the illness, medications, and prosthetic devices out of view of others. Some people go to great lengths to conceal their illness symptoms, even to the point of refusing to seek appropriate treatments. Some others do not even want to belong to self-help groups, probably for fear of discovery. On the other hand, those individuals with symptoms that frighten or repulse others have the most difficulty in normalizing their interactions. Embarrassment, awkwardness, and even rejection prevail. The end result is either limiting interaction to close family and friends or exclusively to persons in similar situations (e.g., self-help groups), or opting for total isolation.

As noted in the previous chapter, one respondent even said that he hesitated to do the interview with me because he did not want other "people to see [him] that way." I did not find anyone with symptoms that frightened or repulsed me, and I wondered how many others there were who would not grant an interview to a stranger because they thought that their symptoms were repulsive. Of course, as mentioned earlier, my data are not representative of all chronically ill people, because I only interviewed people who voluntarily agreed to talk to me. So I probably missed the people who opted for total isolation because they believed themselves to be deformed.

The literature on death and dying similarly demonstrates that it is extremely difficult to keep relationships normal when people know that the illness soon will be fatal. This point is related to what Strauss and colleagues (1975; 1984) termed "identity spread," a process in which most people assume that chronically ill people, especially those who happen to have visible symptoms, cannot act, work, or be like ordinary mortals. Nonsick persons tend to overgeneralize sick persons' handicaps, and these come to dominate the interactions unless the latter use tactics to normalize the situation.

Even if chronically ill persons want to forget the seriousness and fatality of their illness, other people find it extremely difficult to do so and have to work hard at acting normal. One of my respondents expressed this painful fact clearly:

When my hand was so swollen, C. [her daughter] and her husband and her husband's mother and father, and his sister and her husband, we went to a nice restaurant, a German restaurant. The sister and her husband, they seemed like they were afraid to talk to me, like I was, you know, I don't know. The mother talked to me and said about my hand – how swollen it was. But I felt like people thought of me like sort of different because [of my] hand and everything. . . . Yeah, my hand, I had it down. But once in awhile I had to bring it up, you know, well, you know, putting the coat on and taking it off. The mother, when I had my hand up, she always kept looking at it. She had mentioned how swollen it was. Like the sister and the husband, they seemed like, kind of shy, you know, like they thought . . . I was different, you know. Well, I thought why don't they treat me like normal, you know. That's – I read about that most handicapped people want to be treated normal, you know. Like nothing was wrong!

Chronically ill persons in most cases use various normalizing strategies to hide the intrusive symptoms, if possible, or, if not possible, they cognitively reduce the importance of these symptoms to minor status, in order to avoid a stigmatized identity. Normalization processes, then, have behavioral as well as cognitive components and involve many strategies. I identified at least six behavioral and seven cognitive strategies chronically ill people use to counteract the various difficulties caused by the presence of a chronic illness and to normalize their lives.

Briefly, some of the behavioral strategies of normalization are engaging in usual activities despite severe physical limitations, making extraordinary efforts to maintain a normal appearance, pacing oneself or parcelling out energy by giving up certain activities to maintain more important activities, avoiding potentially embarrassing situations, limiting contacts to persons in similar circumstances, and controlling information.

Cognitive components of normalization include minimizing the struggles and adjustments one has to make, being optimistic by saying things could be worse, redefining the normal state as the present plateau of functioning, reordering priorities and values, seeking information that validates personal experiences, engaging in favorable comparisons to similar others who are worse off, and, particularly, engaging in denial of damaging information or new symptoms.

7

Behavioral Strategies of Normalization

Chronically ill persons develop a repertoire of behavioral strategies to assist in normalizing their lives, that is, to continue to live, as much as possible, the way they were living before they became ill, and to proceed with activities and goals as if the illness did not exist or was not an important part of their lives. One way they try to accomplish this is by carrying on as usual.

ENGAGING IN USUAL ACTIVITIES DESPITE SEVERE LIMITATIONS

Many chronically ill people keep the same schedule they met before the diagnosis of their illness, despite exhaustion, the need for extra time for rest to restore energy, and, in many cases, exacerbation of their symptoms. They try very hard to keep up with what they consider normal activities, such as maintaining a job, taking care of household chores, cooking meals, and participating in their usual social events. As a respondent stated: "It's very hard to have a decent attitude toward your health and to also function correctly so that people won't have to keep drawing in on your health and saying she's special. I never once wanted them to say that. I just wanted to say,

"Hey, I can keep it up. For the record, look at my attendance, ten years, perfect attendance." As a result, these chronically ill people suffer the consequences in exacerbation of symptoms, pain, and fatigue. They nevertheless consider these risks worthwhile because t aking them, allows the ill to maintain satisfactory self-images. The same respondent explained:

> The situation the way it was down there [the office] and how stressful it was, I said either I'm gonna learn how to really take care of my health or really take care of my work. You cannot do both, though. I mean, you can't do it. So, obviously, the thing that was most compromising to do, that would be to not take care of my health. It wasn't a purposeful move, it was just the one takes more priority. . . . The health does, and yet I chose to take the other one because it's a normal response.

Some chronically ill people overcompensate, and even engage in what we might call "supernormalizing" to deny incapacity, to prove to others that they are, as one put it, "as good as ever," or to recapture a former identity. A respondent explained it this way:

> Now yesterday, I did something that I probably shouldn't have done, and there was a heavy piece of equipment that we had to take off the truck, and I lifted it, and maybe I didn't lift it right, because my back is bothering me today. You see! But it bothered me all day yesterday, but I can't just say, OK. I'm going to go home today, to relax. . . . Because whatever I should not be doing, I probably do anyway. . . . My boss has been very good to me, and he says, Don't do that and don't do this, get somebody else to do it. After so many years you just can't say I'm not going to do this.

One woman, a long-term sufferer from multiple sclerosis, recalling her younger days, said:

> I was very active, but I really didn't let it get me down too much because I had too much to do. I just have! It didn't put me in bed, it didn't put me in a wheelchair, it just slowed me down. And we managed quite well. My husband worked for a company at that time that was—He was a salesman and we went on a lot of trips,

did a lot of traveling. So, even in spite of the handicaps, we went anyway.

In addition, supernormalizing serves as a tactic to distract ill persons from discomfort and pain, sort of like mind over matter. Another respondent expressed himself this way: "Whatever I could do, . . . to buy a sports car or do golf. . . . It's just to find a way what you can do, what kinds of things you can enjoy. . . . I do things around the house, I try to organize my house. So, whatever I can do and not just keep thinking I'm sick!" An older man discussed his various activities on behalf of his community and church to keep himself very busy so he would not have time to think about his three chronic conditions. He philosophized by saying: "I am the master of my fate, I am the captain of my soul. Now, in that saying that you can keep certain things . . . certain things may happen to you, and you may not be able to handle it, but how you deal with it . . . how you feel, not how to keep it away from you. You may not be able to do that, but how you handle it. Whether or not is up to yourself, and that's all I believe. So, I can deal with it!"

In reality, these people are caught in a serious dilemma. On the one hand, they have to cover up their symptoms so they can keep up with their usual schedules. But on the other hand, they also need sympathy, understanding, and cooperation from those around them when they cannot keep up with their obligations and have to forgo some of their activities in order to restore energy. Nonetheless, these individuals try very hard not only to manage their symptoms and regimens but also to cover up the existence of those symptoms, expending scarce energy to guard against repulsing family and friends and to function in their chosen roles.

Chronically ill persons who get into the habit of covering up most of the time somehow have to provide a rationale to others for not being able to engage in some social activities and sometimes for not being able to fulfill their social obligations. They also have to justify their constant need for extra time to restore energy without letting family and friends know the real reasons for such needs, in order to hold on to their identities as fully functioning adults. Hence chronically ill persons try to normalize their lives by also trying to maintain their former appearance.

MAKING EXTRAORDINARY EFFORTS TO MAINTAIN A NORMAL APPEARANCE

Chronically ill people who want to engage in usual activities despite severe physical limitations, go to great lengths to maintain a normal appearance, no matter what the cost to them afterwards. For example, the woman suffering from multiple sclerosis said:

In fact, I could remember in '65 I wore a brace. I was determined I was going to get out of that brace before we . . . because I had a full back brace. And we were supposed to go to the Bahamas. I said, I am not wearing that back brace on that trip, and I made it. I made my back strong enough so that I could go without it. But even at that time, we'd go walking, then the leg would start dragging, and so I'd have to sit down and rest it. Or we'd be dancing and I wouldn't make it through a whole dance number and all that . . . and that's it. It didn't stop us. We did a lot of traveling. We went to Europe.

Most often, chronically ill persons hide the fact that they are in pain in the presence of others; they maneuver and struggle to normalize social relationships. As one of them stated:

No, I don't discuss things with other people. Maybe that's another one of my problems, but I don't even talk a lot to my wife about these things. My back bothers me? It bothers me! It's my problem! I don't want to tell people: Oh, my back is bothering me today. I gotta take it easy. I don't say these things. . . . Maybe because I don't want them to think I'm weak—you know, that I have to depend on somebody else. I'd rather depend on myself.

Some others, no matter what the cost in time and money, search for the right clothes that would disguise their disfigurements. For instance, one respondent went out of his way and wrote to companies all over the United States until he found a place that would make him a pair of customized plastic braces that he could hide under his slacks and fit into a specially made pair of shoes. He stated that this whole outfit cost him over $1,000 which his insurance company refused to pay, since they had paid for the standard set of metal braces he was supposed to wear. Nevertheless, he felt that this was "a very small price to pay" to keep his problem concealed from others. Another respondent said that even though it is "quite uncomfortable" she wears her breast prosthesis to bed to maintain a normal physical appearance, intended to spare her mate and herself some awkwardness.

Some people also make special efforts to try to normalize their lives by pacing themselves. They seem to parcel out energy by giving up certain activities to maintain more important activities.

PACING

Pacing is an energy-conserving behavior by which chronically ill persons analyze their daily activities so they can balance these activities with needed time for medical regimens and rest periods to conserve energy. As one respondent noted, "For me to do something which I wouldn't ordinarily think twice about doing, but since, you know, I have the asthma, then I have to stop and think, Oh, wait a minute, I really shouldn't be doing this."

Balancing, essentially a survival tactic, is of course, an activity in which all persons are engaged all the time to protect themselves from experiencing the world as intolerably anarchic. Balancing is both a personal activity and, more important, a social process involving negotiation with others as well as ourselves. The same respondent elaborated on the process this way:

I'll be out with my friends and they'll want to do something. Like if they want to go running or swimming and I'm like, OK, we can go, but I have to be careful because I don't want to have any problems breathing. And they're like, OK, no problem, we'll take it slow if you want to. . . . I do go swimming, but when I do I take it real easy and if I feel that I, you know, that I'm having, you know, I'm breathing real heavy, then I stop. I slow down, you know.

For a diabetic, balancing and pacing activities may manifest themselves somewhat differently. For instance, by carefully calculating blood sugar levels occasionally to "cheat on the diet by eating a treat" and then by compensating for it by "being extra good for the next couple of days," a person with diabetes might feel "almost normal, just like being on a diet." Three other interviewees also mentioned using this tactic.

In fact, pacing is desired normalization strategy and results from the way chronically ill persons understand their limitations and abilities and engage in activities over a reasonable time span that can satisfy ego needs without causing undue hardship or exhaustion.   For example, a respondent with cardiac problems insisted that he "can do almost anything" he had done before his illness.   Upon probing, he elaborated by saying that when he feels dizzy, has an upset stomach, or "feels a tightening of the chest," he takes it easy, resting until he can resume his activities.   Another respondent, who perceived being a wife and mother as her desired identity, also paces herself to fulfill the appropriate obligations that she thinks belong with that identity, even though it takes her a lot of time and effort to do so, "I still like to cook but I need a lot of help because I can't cut up things, and, you know, I can't stand for a long time. So anything takes a real effort, you know, a real long time to prepare everything. I still putz around." One respondent mentioned taking three days to do a cleaning chore that once took a morning or afternoon, washing part of her dishes and finishing later, and keeping frequently used items on the kitchen countertops rather than in the basement in order to avoid excessive stair climbing.

Balancing the options, for chronically ill people, includes deciding whether to keep up an activity and suffer the increased symptoms, pain, and fatigue; whether to cover up and risk inability to justify inaction when needed; and whether to elicit help and risk loss of self-esteem or give up the desired activity altogether.

Most of us carry on with our lives based on the notion of an orderly, predictable, and inherently stable world in which plans are made with reasonably confident expectations of their materializing. Predictability, however, is precisely what most chronically ill persons cannot assume.   Accordingly, some chronically ill people use still another strategy to normalize their lives.

AVOIDING POTENTIALLY EMBARRASSING SITUATIONS

Since the uncertainty factor in chronic illnesses makes life more unpredictable for many chronically ill persons and their families, these persons avoid many potentially embarrassing situations. For example, one respondent recalled that she had disappointed her family and friends a couple of times by offering to make Thanksgiving dinner or having Christmas at her house.

> I was feeling pretty good at the time and I wanted to do it. . . . They were always helping me. I love having people around, they love my cooking. But when I started doing it . . . it was too much, I got so sick. One time they had to go out and eat out. . . . I think it was Thanksgiving. . . Another time they had to do all the work, and I could not even help, or eat with them, and I couldn't even sit at the table. They said it was OK, but I felt like . . . So I just don't plan on it, don't offer anymore. I am afraid it's gonna happen again, so I just avoid it.

To avoid potentially embarrassing situations, another respondent, a diabetic, mentioned that she goes shopping when there's nobody around, running back, you still have to look at all those labels. And going shopping is rough, because before I had to take P. shopping going down the aisles and he would, . . . he touched certain things and [would] say, Oh, this is the pop section, right? And, I'd go, Yeah, yeah! And of course, he didn't have enough vision to see, you know, what type or anything. But now I'm finding myself doing the same things that I saw him do. I can see if the letters are large enough. . . It takes me a long time. An older woman commented on the same thing:

> like when you go to a store or something—which I don't do that often. Just those couple times, then, and my hand was so swollen. . . . And I was embarrassed for people to see my hand because it looked so bad. It looked—They do look strange at your hand and talk. They probably think, What's wrong with her? It doesn't make me feel good! You feel like hiding your hand, you know, so they wouldn't look.

Obviously, these respondents do not want to be embarrassed by total strangers staring at them because of their disabilities, so they try to anticipate and avoid such circumstances whenever possible.

LIMITING CONTACTS TO PERSONS IN SIMILAR CIRCUMSTANCES

Since most people, chronically ill or not, would not knowingly put themselves in potentially embarrassing situations, some chronically ill persons, being in greater jeopardy for such occurrences, use the strategy of limiting their social contacts to people in similar straits.

For example, although she does not consider herself a "blind person," a diabetic with "visual malfunction because of her diabetes" mentioned that most of her friends now come from the Lighthouse, which is an organization that teaches blind people to live in their communities as independently as they can. She stated that she associates with these people because "I don't like to be around people that don't at least consider what I'm going through and respect me, respect my situation."

Similarly, the respondent who was embarrassed and hurt by the reactions of some family members at a public restaurant stated that from then on she has not only refused to repeat the experience by avoiding those people and eating out in general, but also by befriending persons in the same circumstances as herself. Thus, besides her daughter and son, most other people she now socializes with are other patients at the dialysis center, particularly since she spends so much of her time there.

Chronically ill people painfully realize that their social world shrinks as a consequence of their illness. The diabetic woman who is gradually going blind perceptively acknowledged that she only hangs around with other blind people because "my choices were limited to begin with."

CONTROLLING INFORMATION OR COVERING UP

The behavioral normalization strategy most chronically ill people seem to prefer, if they can pull it off, is covering up. As discussed earlier, covering up means keeping signs of illness, disability, and pain hidden. It includes not using assisting devices, such as a cane, or other external signs of handicap, such as a wheelchair. In fact, controlling evidence of discomfort, pain, and fatigue is essential for successful covering up, and chronically ill persons expend a lot of effort covering up, not only to maintain a sense of normalcy but also to avoid questions from curious onlookers and to avoid making those around them feel uncomfortable. For instance, a respondent noted:

> If I have to take my medicine — I still don't like for people to watch me take my medicine; you know, you see so many different people at work and stuff, and asking: What are you doing? Do you have . . . ? And then, they go on through this long thing, and at this point, I really don't want to explain it. It's just something right now I have to live with! So, most of the time, if I feel like I'm having trouble breathing, I'll just go, like maybe into the bathroom or somewhere where no one's really watching me and just take my medicine. Just so I don't get bombarded with questions.

I can personally identify with that situation, because I also remember having to carry my medicine in my purse at all times, in case I ran into an unexpected problem. In addition, I used to switch my pills to a bottle marked "vitamins" so that if somebody saw them by accident, I could pretend that they were, indeed, just vitamins.

Covering up is not a form of denial; it is a strategy to keep the symptoms and disability of illness from interfering with normal social interaction. For instance, a respondent suffering from chronic heart illness stated that he does not let anyone know when he has some pain because he "doesn't want anyone to worry." What he really does not want is for people to make "a fuss" over him, which interferes with his self-image and his efforts at normalization.

Covering up allows chronically ill persons to perceive themselves as they would prefer to be perceived by others.

8

Cognitive Strategies of Normalization

When behavioral strategies fail to accomplish the desired results, chronically ill people also resort to cognitive strategies to normalize their lives. In fact, most of these people use several behavioral and cognitive strategies simultaneously. One of their favorite strategies seems to be to minimize their struggles.

MINIMIZING STRUGGLES AND ADJUSTMENTS

Chronically ill individuals try to avoid acknowledging and dealing with the serious nature of their illness by minimizing symptoms and hardships created by therapy and particularly by playing down consequences of their illness. For instance, throughout one interview, the respondent described his symptoms and the limitations imposed by these symptoms on his activities. He then ended the interview by saying, "I have no real physical problem! . . . My sister has the same problem and the doctors told her not to drive, and she does. So, I still play ball!" A young woman who can no longer function independently because she is almost totally blind said, "I just have a disease, that's all. But it's just, OK, it's a malfunction. That's all it is. It's just like my eyes. I don't have a disease in my eyes; it's just they don't see quite right. That's all!" Another respondent, discussing the adjustments he had to make in learning to live with diabetes and blood pressure problems, stated, "I don't think it was that difficult, I didn't think it was that difficult. I never had that serious a blood pressure problem, either. And my diabetic condition was never too bad. Lots of people go in and out of hospitals; I never had that kind of problem." These chronically ill persons, if they can still function in ways important to them, try hard to convince themselves and others that the struggles and adjustments they have to make are minimal, because this tactic makes them feel just like everybody else.

Another respondent used a slightly different tactic to convince himself and others that his problems were "very common" and therefore "no big deal": "Almost every old person you talk to . . . has the same problems . . . some kind of arthritis. Almost every place . . . where it's just so uncomfortable for them, they have to stop and go, that kind of thing. You talk to them, almost any person . . . I talked to, that has some kind of arthritis. Yeah, older people or younger people. Lots of people!" Other people minimize the adjustments they have to make and the hardships they endure by accommodating their treatment regimens within other daily activities, making sure that these regimens occupy a relatively low place in the hierarchy of their multiple roles. For example, discussing time taken for daily treatment routines and time spent for restoring energy, a respondent concluded, "I guess it's something you can live with, without throwing your whole life up, you know. It's not like somebody who loses a leg and you need wheelchairs, you need ramps, you need the same. It's not the same! . . . I'm not saying it's a lot of fun living with it. . . . You can live with it!" The foregoing example also includes the comparison between the respondent's condition and that of those far worse off.

OPTIMIZING (SAYING IT COULD BE WORSE)

The sentiments expressed by the 50-year-old male respondent just quoted is not unusual, since people often use several strategies, such as minimizing and being optimistic, at the same time, to convince themselves and others that it's not so bad, followed by the sentiment that it could be worse. In fact, the respondent who insisted that he had "no real physical problem" because he could "still play ball" followed these comments by saying, "Well, it could be worse; I could be in a wheelchair. That is the ultimate end of the line for my disease."

Furthermore, even if they do not have concrete evidence that others have it worse, some ill persons still try to convince themselves that there must be others who are worse off than they are, perhaps to preserve their self-esteem. As one of the quoted respondents remarked,

> Some people have all kinds of problems, and I sympathize with them. And other people don't have nothing wrong with them, I don't want to say perfect, but they might have something that I don't know about; maybe something mental that they have that I don't have. So, thank God that whatever I got I can live with and suffer along with it. . . . It could always be worse!"

Another respondent was very much aware of the various cognitive strategies he was using to make himself feel good. In fact, he tried to explain the purpose of these strategies to me:

> I use, you know, a little bit different kind of approach. . . . You find out some other means of giving yourself support, because trying to change something you can't makes you feel more depressed. So accept it! My situation probably is much better, probably [than] if I had terminal cancer or something.

A much younger respondent expressed the same feelings, getting right to the point: "I can think of things that can be a lot worse than what I've experienced so far."

Since almost every person in the world, chronically ill or not, can safely make that statement, this strategy seems to be quite popular and effective in making most chronically ill people feel better about themselves and their circumstances.

REDEFINING NORMAL STATE AS THE PRESENT LEVEL OF FUNCTIONING

All chronically ill persons I interviewed had given up some social activities, such as eating out, participating in sports, going dancing, or simply going to some places they used to frequent regularly. But they appeared not to be too concerned about these restrictions and accepted them as part of their present, redefined normal lifestyle. They rationalized, saying that these activities were detrimental to their health anyway, for example, activities such as eating in restaurants. As one respondent mentioned, "You never know what kind of garbage you get for your money in those places. You never know what they put in it or how they prepare it. You're better off doing it yourself at home. And you save a lot of money!"

A younger respondent who used to enjoy meeting friends and drinking in bars regularly said that she really missed not being able to do this at the early stages of her illness, but now believes that

> I've gotten more positive feelings about myself since I have changed my lifestyle around. I think I feel better because I'm in control of my life in general. . . . Calmer, more verbal than I used to be, and, I think when I say more verbal, I mean more assertive and not as aggressive, and there is a difference between the two. I find that there's a more of a creative side of myself than there ever was. If I hadn't . . . had to slow down, who knows, probably, I'd be out running around playing games . . . (laughs) at 32. It's time to slow down!

Some chronically ill persons also accept as normal the symptoms they experience and do not make great efforts toat control their conditions n order to eliminate these symptoms, particularly if they are not too intrusive in important areas of their lives. In other words, if they can function somewhat normally in their chosen social roles, people learn to accept and live with their symptoms without getting too frustrated, since in most cases they cannot eliminate the symptoms, no matter how hard they try. A respon-dent explained his attitude toward continuing symptoms by saying: "To try to indulge too much won't do any good; also, it won't do any good if you try to control it too much. . . . For me, the most helpful advice for this condition is not to forget you are sick. . . . How to exist with your illness, existence is very important . . . to live with it!"

REORDERING PRIORITIES AND VALUES

Whether it is rationalization or realistic appraisal of their situations, most people, chronically ill or not, seem to adjust their priorities and values to correspond to their actual life situations and in particular to their level of functioning, especially if they perceive it as a consequence of the aging process. In fact, most older respondents, in one way or another, expressed a view similar to the respondent who said "as people get older, they cannot do many of the things that they wanted to do anyway, because the body is not what it used to be."

Even younger chronically ill people adjust their priorities and values to their situations and find reasons for doing so, since they have little choice in the matter, under the circumstances. A respondent who had to give up her physically demanding job and many of her enjoyable social activities because of her illness stated:

> And I used to dance quite a bit. And I find that even getting up there for just a couple of songs to dance, it's just very . . . shortness of breath a lot, and I — sometimes it depresses me but, like the last four years, especially discovering I've got a talent for doing crafts and writing and that, it compensates for other things. And, I figure, at 32 it's about time you got off the dancing and found something else you wanted to do with your life, you know [laughing]. And I don't enjoy nursing anyway! . . . After working in a hospital for 12, it's just something I don't want to have to deal with anymore. I don't want somebody else pushing my buttons and setting my hours for me and pulling my little puppet strings. . . . Nursing, especially, took up so much of my time that I never realized I had a creative side. You know, till I was forced to sit down on my backside for a while, and in a way, that is what's good about, you know, having to rest more, and do quiet things more. Then, you realize you can do them . . . it's a part of being me, now. . . . So much for [the] better, I'll sit in my backyard and play with my poem, and that is what I want to do!

In general, I found that changes in enjoyment of life reported by the chronically ill people I interviewed appeared to reflect their attitudes on life before the onset of their illness and their expectations of what they should be doing or be able to do at the current stage of their life despite their illness. For example, a respondent who said that all his life he put the welfare of others before his own, particularly making sure that his kids had everything they needed, including a good education and "things [he] didn't get," felt that at this stage of his life it was time to take care of himself: "I have to think of myself, and I know it's not nice to say you have to think of yourself all the time. But, if I don't think of myself, nobody else is going to think of myself."

Another respondent expressed the same feelings, also with a need to justify these feelings:

> You know, it took me a long time to realize that thinking about me wasn't selfish. . . . For so long, I never thought about me. . . . Since I had her [daughter] it was work around the clock . . . making sure she was fine. . . . For the first 14 years of her life, was just insulin shot reactions and trying to keep her health . . . and then just taking care of her, Oh, it's time for her shot now! Now, it's time for her meal! Now, it's time to cook . . . and my whole life, I didn't have time to think about me, you know? And then, when I realized I had to think about me, I felt guilty. It took me a long time to say, if I don't make me better, who is gonna take care of all of them anyway?

Two younger respondents expressed similar views, but they arrived at opposite conclusions, saying that they were, as one put it, "too selfish, too self-centered," so the illness has made him reflect on his life, and made him "more aware of God," or at least made him become more sensitive to the needs of others around him. Another respondent said:

> It's made me a little bit more aware, I think, of people that might have other problems. Like, I always make sure that people aren't going through the same thing that I am, that I have gone through. . . . So, you know, if someone's out of breath or something, I'll go up to them, you know, concerned. . . and I don't think I'd be as acutely aware of that if I hadn't gone through it myself. . . . I'm very open-minded when things come up, and that might've even been because of the asthma, that I'm a little bit more compassionate, a little bit more open to what other people are feeling, thinking.

Most chronically ill people, however, simply said that they wanted to continue living their lives as normally and as independently as they could without having to worry about inconsequential matters. For example, a respondent expressed these feelings by stating that "I'm learning how to not be bothered by people that I think might be watching me, . . . I'm walking a little differently or that I'm looking a little differently."

Indeed, all respondents, in one way or another, expressed the feeling that having a chronic illness was a significant event in their lives that led them to rethink their attitudes and priorities and forced them to restructure their lives along more satisfying lines. As one of the respondents quoted, summarized:

> It taught me to slow down. I mean, I used to be a very wild individual; you know, I'd be out dancing and carousing and being in the bar so long, most of the night and evenings, flaunting around with kind of a wild crowd. And, it taught me that, Hey! There are other things in life besides sitting in the bar, and you better find out what they are, because you don't have much of a life left. And it taught me that, if nothing else. . . . I'm sorry it took something so drastic to kick some sense into my head, but in the long run, I think it's done me more good than harm at this point.

For most of these people, chronic illness became a spiritual encounter as well as a physical and emotional experience. As mentioned earlier, some of them even perceived the experience as a blessing in disguise. Rationalization or not, this way of thinking undoubtedly helps these people normalize their situations, at least cognitively.

SEEKING INFORMATION THAT VALIDATES PERSONAL EXPERIENCES

A number of studies in social psychological research have shown that people in general, chronically ill or not, seem to need to know that they are not alone in their predicaments, that other people are also going through the same experiences, especially if these experiences are negative. As the popular folk saying suggests, "Misery loves company." Finding out that other people are going through the same experiences makes chronically ill people feel that their situation is a least not that unusual, but is in fact part of the common human experience, and thus normal.

Consequently, these people go out of their way to seek information to validate their personal experiences. For instance, a respondent stated, "I sent away to the Arthritis Foundation. They sent me several pamphlets on arthritis, back problems. And I read articles that people have the same problems and I can read the article and . . . they're all the same. Everyone is the same! Your back goes out, you have to [lie down] 10 days, relax, do your exercise and that's it." Some people exchange information with others in similar circumstances, read everything relevant to their illness in newspapers and magazines, and/or watch programs on television that are related to their health problems.

Others, although very few (only 4 people out of 35), said that they had joined self-help groups. I asked all my respondents if they were aware of the existence of such groups within their area, and more than half indicated that they knew of such groups, but for some reason or another most of them could not exactly explain their reluctance to join these self-help groups. For example, one respondent who eventually joined such a group explained:

Not initially, I didn't, because the idea of going to listen to – I wasn't too big on the idea of going to listen to other people talk about it. I figured it was problem I had to work out myself. It became helpful later on, knowing that there were other people that had it and had basically the same problems. But at first, I really wasn't too big on the idea of going to listen to a group discussion about it, I suppose. I wanted to find out all the information I could myself, and I figured I had to work it out my own way, and that's basically what I tried to do, and it must have been about a year, year and a half, before I went to some of these group meetings. Well, my wife was pushing! She said, Well, we should go and see, and I said, I guess I should, and I says it won't hurt now to go. And, also the fact that they had some good speakers that I wanted to hear. They had people from – they had neurologists, doctors talking, and they had people from the government that would help you, etcetera. Matter of fact, they even had somebody from the IRS talking about the types of benefits . . . I guess what interested me about going initially was the fact that they did have

some good speakers . . . and also, I figured it would be nice to talk
to other people with MS, how they had handled it, how I was
handling it versus how they were handling it.

The three other people from my sample who had also joined self-
help groups indicated that the main reasons they attended, as one put
it, "only a few, maybe a couple of meetings," were to get information
about their illness, to see if they could get some pamphlets, to find out
how to file for disability benefits and to see how other people were
handling illness — and treatment — related problems, in that order.
None of these people continued going to these meetings after a few
times. Another respondent explained why: "I got the information I
needed, they were quite helpful . . . it's a waste of time to sit around
feeling sorry for yourself week after week. You gotta get on with it."
It makes sense, considering all the different strategies people use to
avoid being stigmatized and the various efforts they make to live as
normally as they can, that they would not want to associate exclusively
with other chronically ill people if they could help it. A respondent
who considers her heart condition not too debilitating said, "Joining
a group? No! It's just not incapacitating, or it doesn't bother me
mentally enough, besides the fact that I don't think there are groups
of people . . . as such, you know, maybe for people who had a heart
attack or had bypass surgery and so sign up for their exercise routine
and have gym together or something but—" These people, like others
who may not want to join self-help groups, as those for arthritis and
diabetes sufferers, are mostly concerned with normalizing their situations rather than constantly being reminded that they are chronically
ill people.
Furthermore, when asked to evaluate their coping strategies in comparison with people they met in these self-help groups, the joiners all
indicated that they thought they were doing OK, that they were
handling their problems better than most people they met in these
groups. Since they seemed to believe that they were already managing
better than other group members, it made sense for them not to
continue to attend further meetings.

ENGAGING IN FAVORABLE COMPARISONS TO SIMILAR OTHERS

For purposes of social comparison, chronically ill persons seem to select individuals in the same circumstances who are worse off than themselves. As a respondent suffering from kidney failure remarked:

Well, some of the people are much worse off than I, not all of them, but there is one woman who has diabetes and her legs are all swollen and, I'don't like pus. They're all bandaged up and like pus or something—blood and everything comes through the bandages, and I mean she is in terrible shape. And, there's another one, she had diabetes and also kidney failure . . . and they had to cut her toes off and then they had to take her eye out. I mean when you look at that, you think I'm not that bad off!

Among all the people I interviewed, as noted, not a single person admitted knowing another individual suffering from the same illness who was doing better or coping better than themselves. This finding led me to think that these people either purposely ignored those who were doing better under similar circumstances or, more likely, chose to remember only those people who were doing much worse. For example, a respondent told me that having arthritis was very common among people in his line of business—plumbing and construction work. However, when pressed to come up with a specific example, he said, "I've known several people in the business—at this point, I don't know." He later remembered: "My nephew's wife's mother, his mother-in-law, I would say, had arthritis in her hands, and they operated on all of of them and took out the bone or the calcium, and now she can move her fingers like a person. . . . Well, the ones that I have [known] I guess have rheumatoid arthritis, that's the worst, when the bones are affected!"

Such downward comparisons as "I'm really much better off than she is" (a comment made by a respondent comparing herself to a friend in the same situation) do seem to bolster the sense of self. Indeed, the respondent who made this comment, a woman suffering severely from multiple sclerosis yet leading an active social life as wife, mother, and traveling companion for her husband, proudly declared, "I have a friend who—we met through a mutual person—same age as I am, has four children, and in five years she was in a wheelchair, could not use her legs at all, and could barely use her arms. She was a nurse, she had four young children, and the same situation, identical. She was an ambitious person."

Even if they don't know a specific individual for comparison, chronically ill persons still seem to think that they are doing better, coping better, or in general are better off than others in the same circumstances. For instance, another respondent suffering from arthritis, after describing at length her various difficulties, still concluded by comparing herself favorably to others:

> But, it's such a severe pain, I just, you know, I had two cesareans, I had a hysterectomy, I never ever had pains like this and it's so hard to deal with! If I type, I can't type no longer than an hour at a time. I can't clean house like I used to. I can't bowl. . . . I went to the health club three times a week. The first year when I got off drugs, I gave it up completely 'cause half the times I couldn't get my arms over my head to take my exercises. . . . When I got this in my hand, I had to take all the fluid out of my hand, and fill it with cortizone because I couldn't straighten it up. And I notice now that sometimes when I like sit for too long and I go to get up, it's always my fear, all the way up to ten minutes until I can get—I'm a morning person. I used to jump out of bed, you know, loving mornings. Now, sometimes when I go to jump out of bed, I can't move out of bed, so I sorta just roll out of bed. But, mornings for me aren't as bad as they are for most arthritics! Me, I don't get as stiff!

Furthermore, I noticed that chronically ill people whose adaptations to the illness, or normalization efforts, appear to be more successful than those not as able to adapt well (by their own definitions) choose dimensions of self-evaluation on which they can feel good. No matter how bad things are, these people seem to find an aspect of their situation or a personal characteristic that makes them feel better. As the respondent suffering from multiple sclerosis, still comparing herself to her friend, further elaborated:

> Yes, she got it [the illness] at the same age as me. Now, why did she so quickly wind up in a wheelchair? And really, I didn't wind up with anything. I was still able to keep going. Of course, my mother says I'm so stubborn, I would not stay in a wheelchair.

Because I was in a wheelchair for three months that I was in the hospital . . . And when I came home I was in a wheelchair for a couple of months, but I wasn't about to stay there, if I was able to manage at all. So as soon as I was able to grasp the cane so I'd have support, I was up! Or maybe I had more determination than some people. I don't know.

Of course, some of the beliefs reflected in these processes may be illusionary, based less on fact than hope; yet for people trying to cope and learn to live with ongoing and incurable illness, hope and illusions can pave the way for constructive action that will enable them to go on with their lives. Sometimes, the hopeful illusion continues even when it is not really justified. At the time of the interview, the respondent just quoted was in a wheelchair herself.

ENGAGING IN DENIAL OF DAMAGING INFORMATION OR NEW SYMPTOMS

Quite a few respondents, particularly younger ones, indicated that they really do not want to know the extent and the seriousness of their illness, since they know that their illness is incurable. As one respondent confessed, "I never wanted to accept the problem! I don't pay attention to—I'm trying to fight it. . . . I fight it by staying active in sports. . . . I don't want to think about me getting worse!" Another respondent, talking about trying to ignore her illness as much as she can, stated:

I don't think it will clear up on its own, or heal, you know, and I don't know if you can honestly say that this is a disease, but it's not such a disabling disease that it's going to go, and it's a possibility it could. But if you watch yourself with the way modern medicine is right now . . . so I think drugs, in general are a lot more potent now. . . . And that in a way is better for us because we're able to be more in control of our lives than—So we can control, and that's what's important, I think. . . . You know, I think it's I've lived with it for so long now, that to me it is like a second thing, you know, second nature to me now, and it's there and that's it!

A young woman suffering from diabetes and its progressive complications since childhood recalled, "I think by the time I was 18, I said just inside of myself: I'm going to school, I'm going to work; let's forget this thing!" At present, this respondent can no longer deny having the illness because of progressive blindness and other emerging problems, yet she still tries to put off acknowledging new symptoms as long as she can:

> I didn't expect to have to go through these other changes this year. I didn't totally accept it until I had to. Well, maybe God will give me a miracle, and I think in the back of your mind you're always hoping that. Then I guess it's a miracle I've been alive for all these years with what I have had and I didn't dwell in my skin, you know, not really been sick or anything and I guess, just time to live each day as long as I can, you know, as normally as I can.

Many respondents seem to use this tactic in their day-to-day living by ignoring damaging information about their symptoms as they attempt to achieve a normal but restricted life. Those who constantly worry or agonize about their illness and/or closely monitor their symptoms find that it interferes with their social roles and obligations. They also find that it interferes with their relationships, because other people perceive them as coping poorly with their illness. In fact, Lazarus (1983) points out that denial is no longer denounced as the primitive and eventually unsuccessful "defense" it once was. The idea that normal cognitive functioning depends upon illusion is increasingly gaining support among clinicians and health psychologists, who now recognize its value in protecting people against crises, both in the initial stages of threat and subsequently, when people must come to terms with information that is difficult to accept, such as the diagnosis and prognosis of a chronic illness. Thus the more successful normalizers seem to be those people who are able to use the tactic of denial of damaging information and new symptoms, as much as they can and as long as they can, in addition to some of the other strategies described, so they are be able to carry on with their obligations and relationships in their daily lives as though everything is normal.

Normalization can vary from situation to situation depending on the social, economic, and psychological makeup of the people involved. Because normalization varies from situation to situation, a lot of self-care behaviors on the part of chronically ill people that are perceived to be counterproductive and noncompliant with medical advice are rational and necessary normalization strategies from the perspective of these chronically ill people, given their particular circumstances.

Accordingly, the various strategies people employ demonstrate that the concept of normalization is much more than just another strategy within the process of adaptation to living with a chronic illness, as it has been previously conceptualized by health care professionals and some social science researchers. Normalization is a rather complicated process that has both behavioral as well as cognitive elements involving many strategies. People consciously or subconsciously use many of these strategies, often interchangeably, to learn to live with the uncertainty inherent in chronic illness; they try to overcome or minimize the salient social consequences of their illness, such as stigma and social isolation, in order to get on with their lives.

Indeed, chronically ill people make great efforts despite their illness to fullfill their chosen goals, to maintain their valued relationships, and to carry on with their obligations. In many cases, chronically ill people do these things at great expense to their health, because maintaining their identities as normal, functioning adults is more important to them than anything else, including exacerbation of their symptoms.

Part IV

Crucial Dilemma for Chronically Ill Persons

I believe you have to look reality in the eye . . . and deny it.

— Garrison Keillor

The basic difference between chronic sufferers and relatively healthy people is merely that the former have additional burdens; they must learn to live with their incurable illness, their ever-present and sometimes unpredictable symptoms, and often with their special, costly, and difficult treatment regimens. As a result, the illness becomes the central focus of chronically ill persons' lives. By necessity, everything else becomes of secondary importance, at least initially, in the business of trying to normalize life, to continue to live, to carry on; as much as possible, the way the chronically ill were living before they became ill. In fact, it appears that some chronically ill individuals try even harder to carry on than most so-called healthy people, both because of the threat the illness poses to their self-identity and because of their sense of impending mortality.

Kathy Charmaz (1983) has also suggested that chronically ill people experience a negative sense of self because their illness restricts their activities, isolates them from other people, discredits them by lessening their sense of worth, and causes them to be a burden to others. I found that at the very least, these people try very hard to carry on as well as they can precisely because they want to avoid being a burden to others.

Yet this business of carrying on runs into major difficulties for those with chronic illnesses, who are usually treated within a framework of hospital-based care primarily designed for those with acute illnesses. Under this type of care, help is fragmented, continuity of care outside of the hospital is nonexistent or haphazard, and information to patients about their long-term illness trajectory and diverse treatment methods is often lacking or incomplete. Most of all, since health care professionals, with some notable exceptions (Davis, Kramer, & Strauss 1975; Strauss et al. 1984;) are essentially concerned with controlling symptoms and minimizing physical distress, they fail to deal with the social and psychological factors related to living with long-term chronic illness.

Professionals (physicians, nurses) frequently appear to have treatment goals that are at odds with those of chronically ill patients, since due to their training they usually define illness only, or primarily, in terms of physiological deviations from normal (e.g., sugar in urine, low hemoglobin) and prescribe treatments to manage these abnormalities with little concern for broader aspects of ill peoples' lives. The neglect of social and psychological factors related to living with long-term illness makes care modeled on the acute type highly inadequate for dealing with chronic health problems. Afflicted people have to manage their ongoing symptoms and treatment complications on a daily basis even after the acute phase of their illness is brought under control during their initial hospital stay. In fact, since persons with chronic illnesses generally have to continue their usual social roles and responsibilities in spite of their symptoms and limitations, they cannot assume the sick role past the initial and/or acute phase of their illness. In order to control symptoms, these people need to incorporate the appropriate health or illness behaviors into the context of their daily lives and learn to function and live with their limitations.

Understandably, then, chronically ill individuals define the situation mostly in terms of their quality of life and pay more attention to fulfilling goals related primarily to social functioning (e.g., keeping their jobs, spending time with spouses and children, entertaining friends) than to their physical disabilities.

Brown and colleagues (1981) found that changes in individuals' social activity emerged as the single best predictor of their life satisfaction. Much previous research on the subject was done mostly by health care professionals and had been dominated by a perspective that assumed that physical disability was the main influence on the quality of life of sick and disabled individuals—a view that appears to neglect major determinants identified in the few studies, including this one, of the experience of illness from the perspective of chronically ill persons themselves.

One major determinant, the ability to be productive, is a highly valued trait in our culture. The chronically ill are like most people, socialized—and wishing—to have purpose and meaning in their lives; they want to contribute in some meaningful way to their families and communities. Having a chronic illness does not change internalized values and goals acquired by lifelong socialization processes. On the contrary, it causes reflection on life's accomplishments and an acute realization of the temporary nature of earthly existence.

My data confirm my initial hypothesis that chronic illness assaults peoples' sense of self and brings about a reorganized confrontation with reality. As Moos (1976) noted, there are thoughts of having little time left, especially in comparison with the life expectancies of healthy relatives and friends. Therefore, I also hypothesized that chronically ill persons probably resort to various means to protect their self-esteem and devise all sorts of adaptation strategies to be able to live what they and their significant others consider a normal life.

When I started this research, I originally assumed, apparently as did many other researchers before me, that all strategies employed by chronically ill people were adaptive strategies, that is, day-to-day symptom management styles and/or adjustments to illness demands. But I have found that in addition to such adaptive strategies, the chronically ill also attempt to normalize their condition; that is, in various ways they seem to deny its severity and unpredictability. They also adopt an expressive and cognitive approach solely intended to maintain or renew a positive perception of the self. Thus they achieve normalization rather than adaptation to illness conditions.

In fact, my data show that chronically ill persons take two sets of seemingly divergent approaches toward their illness. On the one hand, they are realistic about their limitations and frankly confront the facts of their illness. They speak about not being able to participate adequately in many of their valued activities and social roles and about accepting their limitations. They describe the necessary adjustments they have to make in their day-to-day living. Many pay careful attention to their bodies, and through testing various approaches, learn what is necessary to keep their symptoms under control and to function as well as they can in important areas of their lives. They also talk about spending a lot of time assessing and measuring their environments so that they can successfully manage to do tasks that are crucial to them. Thus they are adapting to living with illness conditions. On the other hand, mixed with this realistic position is an optimistically positive construction of their situation. I found that chronically ill people engage in various physical and mental maneuvers, such as deemphasizing the extent and importance of their limitations and/or denying the seriousness and changing nature of their symptoms.

These patterns seem to contradict the (Strauss et al. 1975, 1984) "illness trajectory" formulation: "the chronically ill attempt, at every phase, to place themselves somewhere on their trajectory. They seek cues that suggest whether they are moving into a new phase, carefully watching shifts of symptomatology. They may also wait anxiously for the next symptom to appear, debating whether it portends a new phase or whether its presence is only temporary" (Strauss et al. 1984, p. 67). On the contrary, I found that chronically ill persons very often choose to ignore new symptoms rather than waiting for them and debating their significance. In fact, my data show that some of these individuals are so intent on living if at all possible, the way they were before they became ill that they proceed with activities and goals as if the illness did not exist, or they try to pretend that the illness is an inconsequential part of their lives.

In reality, these people are caught in a serious dilemma. On the one hand, they have to cover up their symptoms so they can keep up with their usual schedules. But on the other hand, they also need sympathy, understanding, and cooperation from those around them when they cannot keep up with their obligations and have to forgo some of their activities in order to restore energy. By covering up their symptoms, they do not get sympathy and cooperation when they need it, because others perceive them as trying to get out of their social obligations, as one respondent put it, "for no good reason."

Moreover, by covering up their symptoms and/or not attending to them, particularly by not putting into effect the necessary adjustments in their lives, chronically ill people may be aggravating their illness condition and not getting the needed medical care. Nonetheless, these individuals try very hard not only to manage their symptoms and regimens but also to cover up the existence of those symptoms while expending scarce energy to guard against "turning off" family and friends, all in order to function in their chosen roles. Charmaz (1983) noted that trying to satisfy all the demands is like walking on a tightrope.

Somehow chronically ill persons who get into the habit of covering up most of the time have to provide a rationale to others for not being able to engage in some social activities and sometimes for not being able to fulfill their social obligations. They also have to justify their constant need for extra time to restore energy without letting family and friends know the real reasons for such needs, in order to hold on to their identities as fully functioning adults. Thus, as discussed in the previous section, these chronically ill persons develop a repertoire of behavioral as well as cognitive normalization strategies to deal with all the contradictory needs.

Furthermore, chronically ill persons expend great efforts to try to convey to others the impression that their lives do not significantly differ from those of normal or so-called healthy people. Hence, they, more than average people, seem to engage in impression management, convincing themselves as well, in their efforts of maintenance of self.

Consequently, chronically ill people very often alter their treatment regimens and go against medical advice rather than reduce their social roles or jeopardize their interactions with significant others in their social world. These people, at least most of them, do not deny the reality of their illnesses, but by trying out alterations in their treatment regimens and by exploring the boundaries of their own reactions and the reactions of those close to them, they try to achieve a sense of control over their own lives. They do not deliberately take risks, but attempt to apply the principles of care they have learned from either medicine or their own trial and error experimentations and modify their regimens to fit their desired and valued lifestyles, rather than the other way around. Since illness constitutes only part of their total self, it is a part that most of them try very hard to forget or to push into the background. Yet by doing so, these people are clearly not adapting well to illness conditions and thus, very often, suffer the consequences. Indeed, the price is high, but the role of being a chronically ill person is for them a less salient role in their identity than that of being a husband, a wife, a worker, or a mother.

Thus, normalization versus adaptation has evolved as a conceptualization of a strategic dilemma for the chronically ill, because these two sets of organizing and ongoing strategies often seem to be at odds with one another. Sometimes people make choices in favor of the former at the possible expense of the latter. As a result, the chronically ill are caught between the adaptive need to effect the necessary adjustments in their lives and the normalizing need to maintain their lifestyles and self-concepts.

Indeed, Strauss and colleagues (1984) also seem to be aware of this problem, stating that when symptoms, regimens, and knowledge of disease, including its fatal potential, are very intrusive on social and interactional relations, then ill persons "have to work very hard at creating some semblance of normal life for themselves" (Strauss et al. 1984, p. 79). My study analyzes the various strategies the ill use to make this possible, and it shows that most of these people are so intent on creating "some semblance of normal life for themselves" that they do it even at the expense of their health.

For example, a respondent suffering from diabetes and severe arthritis makes extraordinary efforts each day, no matter how much pain and discomfort she has, to prepare "a home-cooked meal from scratch" for her husband. She also "forces herself" to eat with him, she says, because he does not like to eat alone, feeling uncomfortable when she goes to all this trouble "just for him." Since she knows how much he appreciates a "nice home-cooked meal when he gets home from work," it is worthwhile for her to pretend that she is also doing it for herself, although she aggravates her arthritis by standing "at the kitchen sink so long" and exacerbates her diabetes by "eating stuff [she] should not be eating." This respondent also talked about how much she looks forward to sitting and talking with her husband each evening "just like it should be, as a regular family." Thus she is clearly making a choice between adaptation and normalization, in favor of normalization. It seems that having a normal and pleasant relationship with her husband overrides the additional discomfort and pain she later experiences. In addition, she is taking a serious risk with her diabetes by eating food she should not be eating; in order to keep her relationship as normal as she perceives it to be, she is making the choice not to adapt well to illness conditions. Or it may be that she is doing these things only out of a strong sense of obligation to her husband (i.e., performing a wife's duty) and then justifying her behavior by saying that she wants to do these things anyway. Also, it is possible, in fact probable, that her husband is pretending that he likes these meals and conversations, because it makes her feel good about herself, and thus, going along with the situation, to keep things also as normal as possible. Since I only interviewed the woman and not her husband, this is only a speculation on my part. The point is that whatever their reasons, it seems really important to most chronically ill people to maintain their valued relationships, even at considerable costs.

As another example, a high-level executive suffering from severe coronary heart disease and other related complications, a man who used to "fly around the country constantly to attend important business meetings and play some golf" or "hop to Vegas for a little gambling" has not been able to travel much or do any of the other things he likes so much since he was forced to retire a few years ago due to his health problems. Yet against doctor's orders and despite strong objections from his primary caregiver, his wife, he is still trying to recapture his preferred lifestyle:

> I bought an annual pass for Eastern Airlines and I can go anywhere Eastern Airline goes for a year. I would like to make more, we've made use of it. I would like to make more use of it. It is gonna require an adjustment for her [his wife] because I am going to do things on my own. She is not a person for travel, doesn't like to gamble, and she has problems with – I want to play a little golf, ride bicycles. . . . I'm still type A personality!

Despite the fact that he once ended up in a hospital in Florida for emergency care and another time had to fly home in the middle of a golf tournament because he was suffering from chest pains, he keeps on traveling. Unrealistically, he still invests a lot of money for a yearly pass for airline tickets he rarely uses instead of spending the money for additional care in restful and peaceful surroundings, as his doctors recommend. He mentioned that the doctors think "I'm a pain in the you know what, because I won't listen to them." Obviously, it is more important for him to keep up appearances and maintain his self-image as an independent, dynamic, and physically active person than it is to make the necessary life changes to take better care of his health. His need to hold on to a valued self-image is clearly nonadaptive for his illness condition.

Another respondent, a young man suffering from a degenerative muscle disease (a form of MS) that forced him to quit playing college football, turned down a desk job with good pay in city government offered to him through his family's connections in Chicago politics in favor of two part-time jobs earning a total of less money "teaching high-school kids [to] play ball, plus a job with the park district to coach a womens' basketball team." He says that he prefers these jobs to any desk job, despite the fact that he has a lot of difficulty walking because of the weakened state of his leg muscles. In fact, he cannot even stand up without his braces, and he admits not being particularly crazy about the jobs themselves. He also admits that he is making this choice against medical advice and against common sense, because the more he uses his legs running around, the more pain he experiences. Yet he obviously equates sports, being active, and always doing something with being normal. Throughout the interview, this respondent kept repeating the phrase "I keep active," as though he would go to pieces if he could not remain physically active.

A woman respondent, severely debilitated and presently in a wheelchair from advanced multiple sclerosis, went through two additional pregnancies against all medical advice after she was diagnosed with this dreadful illness, because "my husband and I wanted to have a large family!" Twenty years later, with her kids grown and away from home in college or working, this respondent is still trying to find new ways to normalize her life and maintain her self-esteem by remaining active and productive, despite her symptoms and her wheelchair. As she stated:

> I taught myself to write left-handed. I was right-handed before the MS happened. I do not do much handwriting, I print most of the things. . . . Last semester I went back to school. I went to write, and took a data processing course, and I'm gonna go back in September and take another one. I really was scared, I just didn't know if I—You know, it's been 25 years since I've been back, since I've been at school, and that in itself is scary. Then, to see if

I could get around. . . . I haven't decided if I'm gonna try and do anything with it, but I need to prove to myself that I can do it.

Since she moves with great difficulty in her wheelchair, it would be very difficult for anyone to imagine that she could get a job. Nor does she really need a job for financial reasons, according to her own account, but, as she says "I need to prove to myself that I can do it."

In fact, most chronically ill respondents choose to work even though some of them can manage well enough financially without working and even though working makes their health problems worse, because according to their perceptions having a job means that they are productive, functioning, and normal people. Efforts to maintain the self seem to override a lot of other considerations. However, some chronically ill persons are forced by their employers to retire because these people need flexible work schedules to adapt to their treatment regimens and/or deal with the unpredictable phases of their illnesses. In fact, three of my respondents reported that their employers were either unwilling or unable to make the necessary adjustments in the workplace to accommodate them so that they could continue working. Other chronically ill persons either are too sick to work or have symptoms that interfere with their particular job requirements, but they still try to find ways to lead what they perceive to be productive and normal lives.

For example, another respondent is so severely debilitated from progressive multiple sclerosis that he can no longer work at his job reading blueprints and making tools; his leg muscles have greatly deteriorated and his vision is almost gone. Nevertheless, every day he cares for the family's adopted 2-year-old Oriental child by himself while his wife is out working to support the family. This respondent recounted at length the trials and tribulations he and his wife endured to adopt a child. They could no longer have their own because of his illness, but they "always wanted to raise a family." They were rejected by all adoption agencies to which they applied as poor potential candidates for parenting because of his severe illness. So they went all the way to Korea to adopt a child, and after trials and tribulations there also, they were successful in adopting an abandoned child who has a defective heart valve. Unless operated on in a few years, the child will not reach adulthood. Yet they made the commitment, against all logical advice, to provide the child with all the necessary medical treatments when needed, and endured a lot of difficulty to make the adoption possible. The respondent, in spite of his severe handicaps and his recognition that "the burden on [his] wife was not fair," said that he and his wife feel "lucky and fulfilled" that they have the opportunity to be a family: "We went through the whole thing and we personally feel that there's no reason . . . somebody disabled shouldn't be able to have children or adopt children." Taking care of a small child would tax any 40-year-old healthy adult, not to mention one with as severe an illness as this respondent has, for he has failing eyesight and needs, as he put it "a lot of time off his feet to rest." Yet he is devoting a lot of time, energy, and enthusiasm to taking care of a small child, admittedly neglecting his own physical problems in favor of what he perceives to be a normal family life.

Indeed, as discussed all throughout this book, most chronically ill persons work very hard at creating some semblance of normal life for themselves because their goals are not just to stay alive or to keep symptoms under control but to live as normally as possible, in other words, to carry on as usual despite their symptoms and their illness. Furthermore, some of these people even take extraordinary chances with their health and possibly jeopardize their lives to make it relatively normal life a reality. As the mother of a little girl, a young, married nurse suffering from a degenerative heart condition diagnosed 20 years ago, declared, "If there is anyone who could write a book on 1,001 reasons not to get pregnant, it's me!"

As these and other examples demonstrate, chronically ill people are so intent on living, if at all possible, the way they were before they became ill that they may resort to all sorts of contradictory strategies, take unwarranted risks with their health, and generally proceed with activities and goals as if the illness did not exist. More often, they try to pretend that the illness is an inconsequential part of their existence to protect their self-identities and/or to maintain satisfactory relationships with their significant others. In the process, chronically ill individuals try to balance illness demands against the demands of everyday life, (adaptation) and maintain their personal goals and values (normalization). Succeeding at one usually results in failing at the other. Indeed, in most cases, if they are able to normalize reasonably well, it is at the expense of adaptation to illness demands, because giving in to those demands would result in abandoning a valued role or a cherished activity. Normalization rather than adaptation seems to be the preferred choice, at least among the chronically ill people I interviewed.

9

The Struggle for Identity:
Lessons from the Chronically Ill

People experience life through a self-centered filter.

— Anthony Greenwald

Over the years I have known more than a few people who were devastated by the experience of discovering that they had a serious chronic illness. They were not easily able to accept and learn to live with the limitations imposed by the illness and go on with their lives, not so much because of the medical aspects of the illness, but because of all the social and psychological problems created by the ongoing illness experience. Some of these people became withdrawn and bitter about life in general, giving up on cherished activities and goals and consequently letting the chronic illness control their existence. Yet others were able to survive the initial shock of finding out that they had to learn to live with an incurable, severe, and ongoing illness. These people seemed to be able to "shift gears," readapt to less than perfect conditions, renegotiate their roles, and get on with their lives. Some of these people, in fact, have been able to accomplish more than most people despite their illness, sometimes even against great social and personal odds.

I developed admiration for these extraordinary people, whom I call the "normalizers," and compassion for the people who seemed to have hard lives because of their illness experience. I was interested in the apparent differences among sufferers in terms of adjustment and the experience of learning to live with a chronic illness. Initially, I simply wanted to find out which coping behaviors lead to successful adjustment and/or which ones are counterproductive. As noted, I wanted to get at an insider's view by documenting the experience of living with chronic illness from the point of view of the sufferers themselves. Yet the assumptions of the ill and others around them explaining the success or failure of individual persons living with severe chronic illness concerned me. The emphasis in most of the successful normalization stories, by the people themselves as well as those around them, was on the person's superior intelligence, personal efforts, and motivation. By implication, less successful people were seen as somewhat lacking in motivation, skills, and intelligence. In other words, these people, if not blamed for their problems, were nevertheless blamed for not possessing the necessary qualifications for overcoming them.

My personal experiences and inclinations, coupled with my training in sociology, made me distrust these individual achievement stories and discount the "blaming the victim" accounts (Ryan 1971). For me, as for most sociologists, social barriers are much more powerful than individual shortcomings. Although we cannot help but admire the successful normalizers and superachievers, we cannot endorse the implication that with effort and superior personal qualities, there is no physical problem that cannot be overcome. The physical handicaps and hardships of most chronic conditions are simply not things that can be overcome by endurance, motivation, and personal efforts. As Irving K. Zola (1982, p. 235) so eloquently stated:

> To emphasize individual personal qualities as the reason for success in overcoming difficulties (and the reason for failure if the barriers prove insurmountable) is self-serving for the individual and the society. For individuals who have lost so much, it rewards them at a cost of making them ignore what they owe to some and what they share with others who didn't make it. To the society

this emphasis merely allows the further disavowal of any responsibility, and more important, any accountability, for the process which makes a chronically disabled person's entry or re-entry into life so difficult. Had my family been poorer and less assertive, my friends fewer and less caring, my champions less willing to fight the system, then all my personal strengths would have been naught. On the other hand, if we lived in a less healthist, capitalist, and hierarchical society, which spent less time finding ways to exclude and disenfranchise people and more time finding ways to include and enhance the potentialities of everyone, then there wouldn't have been so much for me to overcome.

Of course, Zola (1982) is absolutely correct. Yet, whatever the circumstances, what distinguishes the people quoted in this book from other chronically ill people, and maybe from most of so-called healthy people, is that these people are the real "copers" and "survivors." They try harder than most people because their lives and identities are in jeopardy. They are people who, while living with additional burdens and daily threats to their lives and self-identities, are still trying to hold on to their lives and identities. As a popular folk saying goes, "They have been dealt a bad hand in the game of life, and they are trying to make the best of it." We might think of these people as superachievers or heros, as we read about them, but I did not get the impression during my interviews that they saw themselves that way. In fact, as Zola would also agree, these are not people who are different from most of us; they are basically people trying to keep on functioning in their chosen social roles, trying not to lose what they already have and value. In short, they are trying to maintain what they perceive to be meaningful normal lives. The fact that they are not giving up and are able to achieve at least some of their goals, in the face of incredible odds, makes them indeed survivors and heros. I came away with a lot of respect for people I interviewed.

In some way I felt relieved to find that these chronically ill people are like most of us; they struggle to keep their desired lifestyles and they work to protect their valued identities as productive workers, husbands, wives, mothers, lovers, and friends just like the rest of us. Sometimes they succeed, sometimes they fail. It seems that the real measure of health is not the absence of disease, but the ability of the individual to function effectively within a given environment. As Ann Landers, a popular newspaper advice columnist, often writes: "It's not what happens to us, but how we take it that counts." Thus, as we watch these chronically ill people, we can see a kind of exaggeration of the problems we all face in the maintenance of self, and we can learn a lot from their example about our own vulnerabilities and daily struggles.

Schlenker (1980, p. 308), in discussing the various reasons people engage in impression management, notes that "social scientists cannot directly observe such private phenomena, but they can make often inferences about them based on other objects or events that they can observe." Schlenker does not think that this should pose too much of a problem for research opportunities, since "social life is replete with pitfalls, pratfalls, and other identity-threatening predicaments. . . . No matter how much thought and effort people expend constructing a desirable identity, they still face the task of trying to maintain the identity when confronted with events that threaten it" (pp. 124–25). Identity has been described as including personal characteristics, feelings, and images as well as roles and social status (e.g., Burke 1980; Stryker 1980; Schlenker 1985), and this is precisely what my study shows. It seems, that the greater the threat to their identity, the more effort people will expend to try to protect it, with whatever means available to them, and even sometimes at considerable cost. This is particularly true for people with strong ego involvement in their identity.

Goffman's (1959, 1967) major contribution to our understanding of the struggle regarding the preservation of the self, which inevitably encompasses self-presentation and social reaffirmation processes that are essential to that preservation, arises from his claim that the self is a sacred object and is more important than anything else to us because it is always with us and represents who we are. According to him, each self is special, and in social relationships, that very special self we have tried to nourish and protect for a lifetime is put on display. Each person has a social mask, a persona, that he or she presents to others. Those others evaluate this mask and make judgments about its appropriateness for playing out or staging the social encounter.

When a person's appearance or behavior communicates some negative meaning, that becomes evidence that the person's persona is not acceptable, as is often the case with handicapped people. Thus the "discredited" person must cope with the consequences of a damaged identity. In the book *Stigma: Notes on the Management of Spoiled*

Identity, Goffman (1963) relates example after example of the various ways in which persons cope with their stigmatized social identities and also how they deal with hidden identities that might be discreditable if discovered. In fact, Goffman (1967, p. 258) states that

> whether an individual is concerned with achieving a personal goal or sustaining a regulative norm, he must be in physical command of himself to do so. And there are times when his aliveness to the contingencies in the situation disrupt his dealings with the matters at hand: his capacity to perform ordinary mental and physical tasks is unsettled, and his customary adherence to standard moral principles undermined.

Goffman adds that "the ability to maintain self-command under trying circumstances is important, as is therefore the coolness and moral resoluteness needed if this is to be done. . . . Society supports this capacity by moral payments, imputing strong character to those who show self-command and weak character to those who are easily diverted or overwhelmed."

Of course, the ability of a person to cope with a crisis situation will be strongly related to socialization experiences that have taught that person how to approach new events in general. Nevertheless, when events occur that breach important aspects of peoples' identity or self-concept, they become distressed and resort to all sorts of strategies to preserve or to restore their identities. Actions and events that catch people "out of face" have impact not only for the actor but also for the interaction and the social structure, because through the lifelong socialization process, people internalize particular standards, construct a self-concept, and become aware of what particular groups of other people require them to be. In other words, they adopt significant others' values, standards, and evaluations as a means of gaining approval, minimizing rejection, and generally maintaining satisfaction and security.

According to both Goffman (1959, 1967) and Schlenker (1980), in order to accomplish this, people consciously or unconsciously attempt to control the images they project because they are always motivated to present themselves in ways that yield enhanced levels of self-esteem and social approval. As Schlenker (1980, p. 307) states, people act to establish associations with desirable images and to disestablish associations with undesirable images, because "images determine how people see themselves and how they are viewed and treated by others. There is invariably some reason for people to control the images they project, since the reward/cost ratios people receive from social life are predicated in large part on these images."

In fact, Goffman (1967, p. 5) stated that "the term face may be defined as the positive social value a person effectively claims for himself by the line others assume he has taken during a particular contact. Face is an image of self delineated in terms of approved social attributes." Therefore, once a particular face is established in an interaction, the actor is committed to presenting a comparable face to the same audience in the future, without identity-tarnishing blemishes. To switch faces is to appear to be inconsistent, which marks the person as one who has no "real" face and thus is not to be trusted to behave predictably in social interactions. For someone or something to challenge the integrity of the constructed self constitutes a real threat, or at the very least creates an embarrassing situation. The discredited person's acute embarrassment is highly discomforting to everyone else, as well. However, Goffman made it clear that maintaining face is not the goal of social interaction; rather, it is necessary background that permits social interaction to continue, because incidents that threaten the face of a participant also threaten the survival of the relationship.

Goffman (1967) has also said that role-specific behavior is based not upon the functional requirements of a particular role but upon the appearance of having discharged a role's requirements. Much of what we call polite behavior consists of an implicit bargain among actors to help one another keep face by not questioning the performances they offer. As noted, a lot of distress is experienced when people perceive their chosen face or performance in a given situation to be inconsistent with the concept of self they try to maintain for themselves and others in that situation. Otherwise, people might not be so willing to take such great care that they act out lines of behavior considered appropriate to their situation or try so hard to at least appear to be in control of their circumstances.

Markus and Wurf (1990, p. 85) state that "the self-concept, of course, is only one of numerous factors, including culture, the social environment, individual need or tension states, and non-self-relevant cognitions, that may directly influence behavior." They acknowledge, however, that "although behavior is not exclusively controlled by self representations, it has become increasingly apparent that the representations of what individuals think, feel, or believe about themselves are among the most powerful regulators of many important behaviors." According to them, "a great deal of social behavior, sometimes quite consciously and sometimes unwittingly, is in the service of various self-concept requirements" (1990, p. 88).

Furthermore, society teaches people to behave consistently. People learn, from very early on, that if they behave inconsistently, they are likely to be punished. One of the major reasons people try to rationalize and manage the impressions they create is to appear as good, consistent people. Normality is the consequence of the management of impressions, according to Goffman (1967). In fact, the more responsible individuals feel for the circumstances they find themselves in or for their own actions, the more they may use impression management to rationalize the behavior or the situation. That may partially explain why people grapple with the "Why me?" question to such an extent and why they attribute negative events and failures to external factors rather than to their own actions.

Whatever their reasons, by manipulating various aspects of their appearance and performance, individuals seek to fashion others' perception of reality. Schlenker (1980, p. 39) notes that "a common occurrence in social life is the attempt to conceal identity-threatening events from real audiences who might disapprove." Hence, through impression management, people try to create an image that will lead others to act as they wish them to act. People, Goffman argues in his classic *The Presentation of Self in Everyday Life* (1959), are deeply concerned with impression management; they attempt to control the impressions they make on others by presenting themselves in the most favorable light. In acting their parts, they are careful to construct their scenery and make use of personal props. Indeed, just as animals have territories that they defend and claim as their own, humans possess contrived and culturally relative, but nevertheless real, senses of territories of the self (cf. Lyman & Scott 1970).

In short, for Goffman (1959), social interaction requires its participants to be able to regulate their self-presentation so that it will be perceived and evaluated appropriately by others. For example, by being careful to wear appropriate clothing for particular social occasions and by presenting a different self in different circumstances, people deliberately use strategies to achieve their purposes. That leads some people to think of impression management, as opposed to expressing one's true inner feelings and beliefs, as a deliberate strategy of manipulation that is phony and unethical.

Schlenker (1980, p. 41) does not agree with that definition of impression management, and states that

> Goffman has often been criticized for paying too much attention to the conscious and deliberate use of impression-management tactics. Although many of his examples do seem to involve such deliberate performances, he acknowledges that impression management is not solely conscious in nature. Performances may become habits or be very useful for impression management purposes while remaining outside the actor's conscious awareness.

Indeed, in choosing which aspect of the self to present in a particular situation, an individual may be choosing among equally true selves. Furthermore, according to Schlenker (1985), as we attempt to influence others' perceptions of us, we often influence how we see ourselves as well. "The boundary between accurate self-presentation and self-misrepresentation further blurs when we realize that people are often taken in by their own performances, coming to believe that they really are the idealized or dramatized identities they project" (1980, p. 39). Thus impression management plays a key role in how we develop and maintain particular identities in our social life. Although people tend to think of lying and manipulation when they think of impression management, it involves other motives as well. The authentic presentation of oneself—trying to show ourselves as we believe we really are—is also a kind of impression management.

In fact, a common goal pursued in social interaction is self-verification—presenting the self as one believes it to be. Indeed, just because people find themselves in identity threatening circumstances does not mean that they can, or want to, discard their lifelong, hard-earned, cherished and nurtured identities or that they are able to change their ways of thinking, feeling, and behaving. As Schlenker (1980, p. 134) states, "actors in predicaments will engage in behavior designed to reduce the potential negative repercussions and maximize their expected reward/cost ratios as best they can, given the nature of the predicament. The more severe the predicament, the greater is the motivation for such behavior." Goffman (1959, 1967) would say that people will go to great lengths to maintain face in front of real audiences.

In sum, Schlenker states (1980, p. 284) that social psychologists are mainly preoccupied "with determining how people *react* when exposed to particular stimuli — how they are affected by the personal appearance of others, for example. Largely ignored is the question of how people *act* in order to establish particular images in front of others, such as by controlling their personal appearances, props, and scenic background. It is past time to redress this imbalance." In this book I have attempted to do exactly that.

Besides having the potential of being useful to health care professionals and family caregivers, this book, as a social psychological inquiry into the meaning of experience, can serve a wider purpose. From examining the extraordinary efforts of the chronically ill, we might also gain new insights regarding ordinary efforts and general tactics people employ in their everyday lives to protect their self-identities.

10

Needed Changes for Health Care

Suffering of some is simply and literally unknown to many in society. This is a special part of reality which, I think is one of our important responsibilities to understand and communicate.

—Alvin Gouldner

In the continuing debate among health care providers, policy makers, medical sociologists, and health psychologists on reforming the delivery of health care, it is necessary to address the social as well as the medical issues relevant to those whose special health care needs have thus far been inadequately met: chronically ill persons.

Traditionally, problems of health and illness were the province of medical personnel, of the doctors and nurses whose training is geared specifically toward curing specific diseases. Indeed, our health care system has been so oriented toward acute conditions and so successful in its efforts both to eliminate diseases (e.g., polio, smallpox, diphtheria) and to provide intensive care in medical emergencies (e.g., trauma, myocardial infarction) that chronic illness has historically not been considered particularly worthy of high-profile attention. Chronic illnesses are by definition beyond the realm of traditional medical science, which has focused on "cure."

At present, relatively little is known about how to prevent and cure most chronic illnesses particularly heart disease, cancer, and stroke, the three leading causes of disability and death in our society. Other chronic illnesses such as arthritis, diabetes, and renal failure, to name a few, also provoke considerable sickness, disability, damage to self-identity, and economic loss. Thus what can be medically accomplished for people suffering with chronic conditions is, in common parlance, mainly "checking the progress of the disease," "getting them on their feet," and "slowing down the inevitable," on an individual basis, rather than curing these people or preventing them from getting ill in the first place.

However, even if we were medically doing all we could and trying as hard as we might, individual efforts would not always be successful in solving the problems associated with chronic illness. These medical efforts, as crucial as they are, need to be supplemented with effective structural changes in how health care is delivered and with social interventions targeted to particular problems experienced by chronically ill individuals. A big part of the problem is the lack of fit between the needs of the chronically ill and the trends and practices in acute care facilities.

Clearly, the medical model, with its individualistic and reductionistic thinking, and the home care system that has fashioned itself on this model, have limitations for chronic illness care. The basic premises of the medical model are that patients are biological organisms and disease is an external threat to be cured (Roth & Harrison 1991). While this model might be appropriate within the context of acute illness, it is not useful for the management of chronic illness. In fact, it is inconsistent with the needs of a society with many chronically ill members, some of them aged and frail, who need supportive services to maintain their lifestyles and their independence. Chronically ill individuals need a health care delivery system sensitive to patient experiences and perceptions. As it is, the needs of most chronically ill people are not being met by the present health care structure. We need a system in which patients are taught how to care for themselves, caregivers are taught how to provide care, and both learn how to access needed services.

In a society where most people, men and women, have to work for wages outside their homes, there is virtually no one available to take care of sick and elderly people on a daily basis. Most chronically ill persons, particularly younger people, have no choice but to work and at the same time manage their illnesses in the context of their lives. As mentioned earlier, the difference between chronically ill people and so-called healthy people is that the former have additional burdens; their goals and desires to remain active and involved in their valued life activities do not change after they become ill. In fact, I found that the actual severity of the illness appears to be unrelated to a person's ability to remain involved in valued pursuits. As my respondents indicated, people will go to great lengths to maintain their desired lifestyles in spite of their illness. Thus health care professionals must take the social and psychological factors related to living with long-term illness into consideration when treating such patients. A health care system that focuses only on medical aspects, ignoring peoples' concerns with issues about their quality of life, is not much help to these people.

Traditionally, there was also a notable blurring of definitions among conditions of chronic illness, disability, and long-term care. Presently we recognize that not all individuals who are chronically ill are functionally disabled, many disabled persons do not require any significant amount of health care, and most chronic illnesses do not require long-term care in an institution, even though these conditions cannot be cured. Furthermore, health care delivery systems are constantly changing, and since most of the daily management of chronic illness actually takes place in the home and is performed by ill persons themselves, a lot of the day-to-day problems these people and their families face are invisible to health care providers. Therefore, it is crucial to take into consideration chronically ill peoples' experiences and perceptions of the situation together with those of health care professionals, in order to get at a more realistic understanding of the total experience of living with an ongoing illness.

Because of the primary importance people place on their quality of life and the recognition that many diseases cannot be cured but only managed, contributions from many other disciplines have been acknowledged, and the field of *behavioral medicine* has developed. Behavioral medicine, started by social psychologists, is an interdisciplinary field integrating behavioral and biomedical science concerned with the application of knowledge to the prevention, diagnosis, and treatment of illness, particularly long-term chronic illness. Social psychologists, particularly health psychologists, are not alone in contributing to this field, yet their contributions—both actual and potential—are considerable, ranging from analysis of the causes of illness, and recognition of patients' perceptions of their illness and treatment to the procedures whereby services are delivered (Taylor 1978).

In fact, there is a tremendous amount of information in the social psychological literature relevant to understanding illness and its treatment. Social psychology deals with the individual within the social structure, examining how that individual interprets what goes on in the environment and how the individual interacts with the social structure to promote her or his values and goals. At the very least, social psychological research contributes in the area of illness management by helping us examine peoples' reactions to illness. Since people have to deal with chronic conditions over long periods of time, it is important for us to know how they feel about their illness, to what they attribute their illness, and how they recognize and interpret changes in their condition. The control and attribution literatures are particularly relevant in helping us understand illness behavior, because these literatures tell us that people act according to their perceptions.

At the minimum, people suffering from life-threatening illness need better methods of controlling pain and discomfort. This is absolutely essential to successful adjustment, because constant pain and/or discomfort affects virtually every aspect of their lives. Indeed, it is hard to think or function well while experiencing bodily discomfort and pain. Everything else becomes secondary to finding ways of alleviating the suffering. While primary advances in pain management have come from medicine, research clearly shows that attributions regarding the nature and cause of pain and discomfort influence how they are experienced. For instance, people are better able to withstand both pain and unpleasant medical procedures when they have clear expectations about the nature of the sensations they can expect and some steps they can take to control the pain (Corah & Boffa 1970). In fact, the actual experience of symptoms may be reduced by feelings of control. There are strong indications, then, that in the area of treatment and management, helping people to control both their reactions to symptoms and their reactions to medical interventions is one of the main areas in which social psychological research has made important contributions. The control literature, especially that on developing appropriate expectations regarding physical sensations as well as that on developing successful coping mechanisms, has been of great help (Langer, Janis, & Wolfer 1975).

In fact, identification of a medical problem requires at least three steps: (1) the prospective patient must recognize that there is a problem and seek medical help, (2) the medical personnel must make a correct diagnosis, and (3) medical personnel must convey this information to the patient and make sure the patient understands what is involved, so that, ideally, caregiver and patient together can decide on and implement a treatment plan.

The traditional "medical model" suggests that there is a recommended treatment or procedure that will cure or alleviate almost any illness. Yet the success of a treatment often depends on the willingness of the patient, especially the chronically ill patient, who most of the time is not under the direct supervision of health care personnel, to comply with the prescribed regimen — to take the pills, show up for chemotherapy or dialysis treatments, observe dietary restrictions, and the like. An important task of the medical practitioner, then, is to convey information to the chronically ill person — information that presumably will affect the person's compliance. Krantz, Grunberg, and Baum (1985) found that in general, the more satisfied patients are with the quality of their communication and interaction with their physicians, the more likely they are to comply with the recommended treatments. Yet too often physicians volunteer too little or no information and the patient asks too few questions, with the result that the potential treatment program encounters real problems (DiMatteo & DiNicola 1982), with negative consequences for care and management of illness. For example, a doctor who maintains contact with families rather than just individuals can more easily understand the many different ways in which people think, feel, and act and the importance of values in medical decision making. Indeed, a doctor who treats chronically ill people, regardless of specialty, needs to be a bit of a family doctor as well.

There is still another advantage in applying the social psychological perspective to issues of health and illness. Social psychology has an orientation to situational variables that elicit, maintain, and control

behavior, thus enabling us to steer away from dispositional explanations for both patient and caregiver behaviors. Indeed, we know from
attributional research that differences between the actor's and the
observer's biases in attribution contribute to misunderstanding between
chronically ill people and their caregivers. Indeed, health care professionals and lay caregivers, like any other observers, would be likely
to show a strong bias toward dispositional interpretations.   For
instance, patients not taking their medications are usually viewed as
uncooperative by their caregivers. Chronically ill people, on the other
hand, certainly have valid reasons for stopping medication if it does
not help or it makes them feel worse. In fact, the side effects of some
medications and treatments are so severe that blindly accepting them
makes any semblance of "normal" existence virtually impossible.
Thus health care professionals and chronically ill persons see the same
event from two different perspectives, and each attends to a different
set of cues. Some of the cues available to one are unavailable to the
other. Besides, their interpretive frameworks are different, and these
differences can have negative consequences for chronically ill people.
Consequently, there seems to be a lot of blaming going around.
Health care professionals blame patients for "noncompliance" instead
of finding out their patients' particular circumstances. As the data
collected for this research indicate, a lot of what appears to be
noncompliance is in fact a normalization strategy on the part of the
patient. Chronically ill persons are indeed caught between "a rock and
a hard place"; they are caught between the adaptive need to effect the
necessary adjustments in their lives because of their illness and the
normalizing need to maintain their lifestyles and self-concepts.
     There is also evidence for patient blaming supported by the "just
world" hypothesis, in which people have a need to believe that victims
get what they deserve and deserve what they get, particularly people
suffering from certain illnesses (e.g., cancer, heart disease, and, most
notably, AIDS). Indeed, since having any one of these illnesses is
regarded as an extremely undesirable fate, well individuals, including
health care professionals and family members, are strongly motivated
to protect themselves by attributing the illness either to sufferers'
undesirable personal characteristics, their past behavior, or their
present inadequacies. Such reactions toward people suffering from
cancer, heart disease, or any other chronic condition are
understandable, because they serve to absolve the blamer from any

guilt about not being able to help or not wanting to help the suffering person.

However, before we ourselves pass judgment on the blamers, we must realize that chronic health problems have enormous consequences not only for ill persons but also for their families, who in most instances have no choice but to assume the role of care provider for extended periods of the family life cycle. Thus, the burden of caring for a chronically ill family member usually taxes immediate family members emotionally, physically, and financially, making the process of trying to normalize the situation very difficult not only for the ill person but for everybody involved.

As a matter of fact, my examination of the various normalizing tactics people employ brought out the fact that chronic illness cannot be managed effectively without taking into account ill persons' relationships with their significant others. Indeed, in many cases family and friends need to act as various kinds of agents: protective, assisting, controlling, redesigning or "covering" in interaction, and the like. Sometimes these people do these jobs very well; other times, for a variety of reasons, they refuse to do them. Yet how they perform as agents may make all the difference in whether chronically ill persons can lead relatively normal lives, whether they grow better or worse, or even whether they survive for very long. In many cases, those in close proximity to people with chronic illnesses try to offer reassurances or even make sacrifices in their own lives to help in various ways, but they become frustrated if they notice little or no improvement in these peoples' conditions as a result. Thus attributing ill persons' feelings and fears to the afflicted persons' personal inadequacy, particularly inadequacies in coping with the illness, can relieve those family members and health care professionals who have frequent and continuing contact with these people from any personal responsibility for being unable, or sometimes even unwilling, to help.

Although there has not been much empirical research on this issue, a number of descriptive studies corroborate this reasoning (e.g., Kalish 1977). Data from my research also support this finding, albeit indirectly. Many respondents made allusions to the effect, that they felt blamed and expressed their frustrations with being held responsible, even by their professional caregivers, for the lack of improvements in their condition. As one respondent, describing her doctor's disapointment with a treatment that did not work, said, "I found myself apologizing to him as though it was my fault! He kept asking me questions and acting as though he didn't believe I did what he told me to do. I should have been the one to be disappointed or angry!" As a result, chronically ill people have the additional burden of trying to convince those around them that the progressive deterioration of their illness is due to circumstances beyond their control and occurs in spite of their many efforts to gain some mastery over the trajectory of the illness.

Indeed, patients are angry or disturbed about what they perceive as "noncaring and judgmental attitudes" of their caregivers, particularly their doctors, without realizing the structural and financial impediments under which individual doctors have to practice medicine. Part of the problem is that more and more chronically ill patients are seen as creating a financial and caseload crisis in hospitals and in an overburdened health care system in general. This group of patients are unpopular with both physicians and hospital administrators. They also strain the already diminishing supply of nurses, because their health care and related needs are constant. Some of these needs are beyond the training, capabilities, and responsibilities of medical professionals.

To be fair, as chronic illness has become our major health problem, its physical, social, and psychological consequences have been increasingly recognized, and a number of specific programs have been initiated to deal with particular problems. Yet at the present time, these programs are not systematically coordinated or widely available to the majority of chronically ill persons. As Relman (1990) states:

> What our health care system needs now is not more money, but different incentives and a better organization that will enable us to use available resources in a more equitable and efficient manner to provide necessary services for all who need them. We can afford all the care that is medically appropriate according to the best professional standards. We cannot afford all the care a market-driven system is capable of giving. (p. 913)

A chief goal for health care professionals, social psychologists, and health psychologists in the coming years, then, should be to help develop programs and cost-effective interventions to improve the quality of life of chronically ill persons and their families.

A first task should be the coordination, identification, and mobilization of existing services within a community so that chronically ill persons and their families can be referred to them when appropriate. A second task should concentrate on making sure that the needed services are available in every community. A third and more important task should involve instituing a standardized and structured system of health care by which an initial assessment of needs in all domains of a patient's life is made right after the patient is diagnosed with a particular chronic illness, during the initial acute period of that illness.

Of course, the initial assessment must be supplemented with regular needs assessment over the long term to identify potential problems, such as depression, anxiety, gaps of knowledge, and difficulties with compliance, before they fully disrupt a patient's life. Systematic and regular assessment, in turn, can help define further the needs of the chronically ill, pointing to new services that may need to be developed. The main purpose of such a system would be to help develop cost-effective interventions to prevent costly and disruptive acute episodes and to improve quality of life for chronically ill people and their families. A network of home—and community-based care as an alternative to hospital care can bring about healthier patients, fewer problems, fewer hospitalizations, and fewer drugs—with a more cost-effective result.

Changing patterns of disease make it necessary to go beyond the traditional biomedical model of health (Krantz, Grunberg, & Baum 1985). Indeed, the extent to which people are able to manage the consequences of chronic illness to lead relatively normal lives depends upon factors ranging across the biological, psychological, interpersonal, economic, and sociocultural spheres of life.

Bibliography

Albrecht, G., V. Walker and J. Levy. 1982. "Social Distance from the Stigmatized." *Social Science and Medicine* 16:1319–27.

Alonzo, A. 1979. "Everyday Illness Behavior: A Situational Approach to Health Status Deviations." *Social Science and Medicine* 13A:397–404.

American Cancer Society. 1989. *Cancer Facts and Figures.* Atlanta, GA: Author.

American Diabetes Association. 1986. *Diabetes: Facts You Need to Know.* Alexandria, VA: Author.

American Heart Association. 1988. *Heart Facts.* Dallas, TX: American Heart Association.

Antonovsky, A. 1979. *Health, Stress, and Coping.* San Francisco: Jossey-Bass.

Arnaud, S. 1959. "Some Psychological Characteristics of Children of Multiple Sclerotics." *Psychiatry in Medicine* 21:8–22.

Atchley, R. C. 1985. *Social Forces and Aging.* 4th ed. Belmont, CA: Wadsworth.

Bagley, C. 1971. *The Social Psychology of the Epileptic Child.* London: Routledge and Kegan.

Barksky, A. J. III. 1976. "Patient Heal Thyself: Activating the Ambulatory Medical Patient." *Journal of Chronic Disease* 29:585–97.

Baumeister, R. F. 1982. "A Self-Presentational View of Social Phenomena." *Psychological Bulletin* 91:3–26.

Birenbaum, A. 1970. "Managing a Courtesy Stigma." *Journal of Health and Social Behavior* 12:196–206.

Birenbaum, A. 1971. "The Mentally Retarded Child in the Home and the Family Life Cycle." *Journal of Health and Social Behavior* 12:55–65.

Bluebond-Langner, M. 1978. *The Private Worlds of Dying Children.* Princeton, NJ: Princeton University Press.

Blumer, H. 1962. "Society as Symbolic Interaction." In *Human Behavior and Social Processes: An Interactionist Approach,* ed. A. M. Rose. London: Routledge and Kegan.

Blumer, H. 1969. *Symbolic Interactionism.* Englewood Cliffs, NJ: Prentice Hall.

Bosk, C. L. 1979. *Forgive and Remember: Managing Medical Failure.* Chicago: University of Chicago Press.

Braden, C. J. 1990. "A Test of the Self-Help Model: Learned Response to Chronic Illness Experience." *Nursing Research* 39:42-47.

Braham, S., H. B. Houser, A. Cline, and M. Posner. 1975. "Evaluation of the Social Needs of Nonhospitalized Chronically Ill Persons: One Study of Forty Seven Patients with Multiple Sclerosis." *Journal of Chronic Diseases* 28(7-8):401–19.

Brown, J. S., M. E. Rawlinson, and N. C. Hilles. 1981. "Life Satisfaction and Chronic Disease: Exploration of a Theoretical Model." *Medical Care.* 19, no. 2:1136–46.

Buchanan, D., and H. Abram. 1975. "Psychological Adaptation to Hemodialysis." *Dialysis and Transplantation* 1:36–41.

Burke, P. J. 1980. "The Self: Measurement Requirements from an Interactionist Perspective." *Psychology Quarterly* 43:18–29.

Burkhart, M. A., and M. G. Nagai-Jacobson. 1985. "Dealing with Spiritual Concerns of Clients in the Community." *Journal of Community Health Nursing.* 2:191.

Callahan, E. M., S. Carroll, P. Revier, Sr., E. Gilhooly, and D. Dunn. 1966. "The Sick Role in Chronic Illness: Some Reactions." *Journal of Chronic Disease* 19:883–97.

Carlson, C. 1979. "Conceptual Style and Life Satisfaction Following Spinal-Cord Injury." *Archives of Physical Medicine and Rehabilitation* 60:346–52.

Carver, C. S. 1979. "A Cybernetic Model of Self-Attention Processes." *Journal of Personality and Social Psychology* 37:1251–81.

Charmaz, K. 1983. "Loss of Self: A Fundamental Form of Suffering in the Chronically Ill." *Sociology of Health and Illness* 5:168–95.

Charmaz, K. 1987. "Struggling for a Self: Identity Levels of the Chronically Ill." In *Research in the Sociology of Health Care: The Experience and Management of Chronic Illness,* ed. Juluis A. Roth and Peter Conrad, 283–321. Greenwich, CT: JAI Press.

Charmaz, K. 1991. *Good Days Bad Days: The Self in Chronic Illness and Time.* New Brunswick, NJ: Rutgers University Press.

Chirisman, N. 1977. "The Health Seeking Process: An Approach to the Natural History of Illness." *Culture, Medicine, and Psychiatry* 1:351–77.

Christopherson, L., and T. Gonda, 1973. "Patterns of Grief: End-Stage Renal Failure and Kidney Transplantation." *Transplantation Proceedings* 5:1051–57.

Cicourel, A. V. 1974. *Cognitive Sociology.* New York: Macmillan.

Cockerham, W. C. 1981. *Sociology of Mental Disorder.* Englewood Cliffs, NJ: Prentice Hall.

Cogswell, B., and D. Weir. 1973. "A Role in Process: Development of Medical Professionals' Role in Long-Term Care of Chronically Diseased Patients." *Journal of Health and Human Behavior* 5:95–106.

Cohen, F., and R. S. Lazarus. 1983. "Coping and Adaptation in Health and Illness." In *Handbook of Health, Health Care and Health Professions,* ed. D. Mechanic, 608–35. New York: Free Press.

Cole, P. 1979. "Morbidity in the United States." In *Patients, Physicians and Illness,* ed. E. G. Jaco. New York: Free Press.

Commission on Chronic Illness. 1956. In *Guides to Action on Chronic Illness,* ed. L. Mayo, 9–13, 35, 55. New York: National Health Council.

Consumer Reports. 1990. "The Crisis in Health Insurance: Who Loses It? What Happens?" *Consumer Reports* 55, No. 8: 533–49.

Corah, N. L. and J. Boffa. 1970. "Perceived Control, Self-Observation, and Response to Aversive Stimulation." *Journal of Personality and Social Psychology* 16:104.

Corbin, J. M., and A. Strauss. 1988. *Unending Work and Care.* San Francisco, CA: Jossey-Bass.

Coughlan, A. K., and M. Humphrey. 1982. "Presenile Stroke: Long-Term Outcome for Patients and Their Families." *Rheumatology and Rehabilitation* 21:115–22.

Croog, S. 1981. *Life After a Heart Attack.* New York: Human Sciences.

Croog, S., and E. F. Fitzgerald. 1978. "Subjective Stress and Serious Illness of a Spouse: Wives of Heart Patients." *Journal of Health and Social Behavior* 19:166–78.

Darling, R., and J. Darling. 1982. *Children Who are Different: Meeting the Challenges of Birth Defects in Society.* St. Louis: C. V. Mosby.

Davis, F. 1963. *Passage Through Crisis.* Indianapolis, IN: Bobbs-Merrill.

Davis, M. 1973. *Living with Multiple Sclerosis.* Springfield: Charles C. Thomas.

Davis, M. Z., M. Kramer, and A. L. Strauss. 1975. *Nurses in Practice.* St. Louis: C. V. Mosby.

DeNour, A., J. Shaltiel, and J. Czaczkes. 1968. "Emotional Reactions of Patients on Chronic Hemodialysis." *Psychosomatic Medicine* 30:521–33.

DePaulo, B. M. Brown, S. Ishii, and J. D. Fisher. 1981. "Help that Works: The Effects of Aid on Subsequent Task Performance." *Journal of Personality and Social Psychology* 41:478–87.

Deutscher, I. 1973. *What We Say/What We Do: Sentiments and Acts.* Glencoe, IL: Scott, Foresman.

Diller, L. 1976. "A Model of Cognitive Retraining in Rehabilitation." *Journal of Clinical Psychology* 29: 74–79.

DiMatteo, M. R., and D. D. DiNicola. 1982. *Achieving Patient Compliance: The Psychology of the Medical Practitioner's Role.* New York: Pergamon.

Dimond, M. 1979. "Social Support and Adaptation to Chronic Illness: The Case of Maintenance Hemodialysis." *Research in Nursing and Health* 2:101–8.

Dimond, M. 1980. "Patient Strategies in Managing Maintenance Hemodialysis." *Western Journal of Nursing Research* 2:555–74.

Dimond, M., and S. L. Jones. 1983. *Chronic Illness Across the Life Span.* Norwalk, CT: Appleton-Century Crofts.

Dreitzel, H. P. 1970. *Recent Sociology No. 2: Patterns of Communicative Behavior.* New York: Macmillan.

Dubois, R. 1959. *Mirage of Health.* New York: Harper and Row.

Estes, C. L., and L. E. Gerrard. 1979. "Social Research in Health and Medicine: A Selected Bibliography." In *Handbook of Medical Sociology,* 3rd ed., ed. H. Freeman, S. Levine, and L. Reeder. 475–504. Englewood Cliffs, NJ: Prentice Hall.

Fagerhaugh, S. Y., and A. R. Strauss. 1977. *Politics of Pain Management.* Reading, MA: Addison-Wesley.

Farina, A., C. H. Holland, and K. Ring. 1966. "Role of Stigma and Set in Interpersonal Interaction." *Journal of Abnormal Psychology* 71:421–28.

Feldman, D. J. 1974. "Chronic Disabling Illness: A Holistic View." *Journal of Chronic Disease* 27:287–91.

Festinger, L. 1954. "A Theory of Social Comparison Process." *Human Relations* 7:117–40.

Fisher, J. D. and A. Nadler. 1974. "The Effect of Similarity between Donor and Recipient on Recipient's Reactions to Aid." *Journal of Applied Social Psychology 4(3): 230–43.*

Fishman, D. B. and C. J. Schneider. 1972. "Predicting Emotional Adjustment in Home Dialysis Patients and Their Relatives." *Journal of Chronic Disease* 25:99–109.

Fox, R. C. 1957. "Training for Uncertainty." In *The Student-Physician: Introductory Studies in the Sociology of Medical Education,* ed. Robert K. Merton, George C. Reader, and Particia Kendall, pp. 207–41. Cambridge, MA: Harvard University Press.

Fox, R. C. 1959. *Experiment Perilous.* New York: Free Press.

Fox, R. C. 1980. "The Evolution of Medical Uncertainty." *Milbank Memorial Fund Quarterly/Health and Society* 58, no. 19 (Winter).

Fox, R. C. 1989. *The Sociology of Medicine: A Participant Observer's View.* Englewood Cliffs, NJ: Prentice Hall.

Freidson, E. 1960. "Client Control and Medical Practice." *American Journal of Sociology* 65:374–82.

Freidson, E. 1965. "Disability as Social Deviance." In *Sociology and Rehabilitation,* ed. M. Sussman. Washington, DC: American Sociological Association.

Gallagher, E. B. 1976. "Lines of Reconstruction and Extension in the Parsonian Sociology of Illness." *Social Science and Medicine* 10:207–18.

Garfinkel, H. 1967. *Studies in Ethnomethodology.* Englewood Cliffs, NJ: Prentice Hall.

Garrity, T. 1973a. "Social Involvement and Activeness as Predictors of Morale Six Months after First Myocardial Infarction." *Social Science and Medicine* 7:199–207.

Garrity, T. 1973b. "Vocational Adjustment after First Myocardial Infarction: Comparative Assessment of Several Variables Suggested in the Literature." *Social Science and Medicine* 7:705–17.

Glaser, B. G., and A. L. Strauss. 1966. *Awareness of Dying.* Chicago: Aldine.

Glaser, B. G., and A. L. Strauss 1967. *The Discovery of Grounded Theory.* Chicago: Aldine.

Glaser, B. G., and A. L. Strauss. 1968. *Time for Dying.* Chicago: Aldine.

Goffman, E. 1959. *The Presentation of Self in Everyday Life.* Garden City, NY: Doubleday Anchor.

Goffman, E. 1961. *Asylums: Essays on the Social Situation of Mental Patients and Other Inmates.* Chicago: Aldine.

Goffman, E. 1963. *Stigma: Notes on the Management of Spoiled Identity.* Englewood Cliffs, NJ: Prentice Hall.

Goffman, E. 1967. *Interaction Ritual: Essays on Face-to-Face Behavior.* New York: Doubleday.

Goldberg, R. 1974. "Vocational Rehabilitation of Patients on Long-Term Hemodialysis." *Archives of Physical Medicine and Rehabilitation* 55:60–65.

Gordon, G. 1966. *Role Theory and Illness.* New Haven, CT: College and University Press.

Gordon, W., I. Freidenberg, L. Diller, L. Rothman. 1977. "The Psychosocial Problems of Cancer Patients: A Retrospective Study." Paper presented at the American Psychological Association meeting in San Francisco, CA.

Gouldner, A. 1973. *For Sociology.* London: Allen Lane.

Greenberg, M. S. 1980. "A Theory of Indebtedness." In *Social Exchange: Advances in Theory and Research,* ed. K. J. Gergen, M. S. Greenberg, and R. H. Willis. New York: Plenum.

Gussow, Z. 1964. "Behavioral Research in Chronic Disease: A Study of Leprosy." *Journal of Chronic Disease* 17:179–89.

Gussow, Z., and G. S. Tracey. 1968. "Status, Ideology and Adaptation to Stigmatized Illness: A Study of Leprosy." *Human Organization* 27, no.4:316–25.

Haber, L. D. 1971. "Disabling Effects of Chronic Disease and Impairment." *Journal of Chronic Disease* 24:469–87.

Haber, L. D., and R. Smith. 1971. "Disability and Deviance: Normative Adaptations of Role Behavior." *American Sociological Review* 36:87–97.

Hakmiller, K. L. 1966. "Threat as a Determinant of Downward Comparison." *Journal of Experimental Social Psychology Supplement* 1:32–39.

Haynes, R. B., M. E. Mattson, A. V. Chobanian, J. M. Dunbar, T. O. Engebretson, T. F. Garrity, H. Leventhal, R. J. Levine, and R. Levy. 1982. "Management of Patient Compliance in the Treatment of Hypertension." *Hypertension* 4:415–523.

Health Care Financing Administration. (Nov. 18) 1988. Washington, DC: Government Printing Office.

Hilton, B. A. 1988. "The Phenomenon of Uncertainty in Women with Breast Cancer." *Issues in Mental Health Nursing* 9:217–38.

Holcomb, J., and R. MacDonald. 1973. "Social Functioning of Artificial Kidney Patients." *Social Science and Medicine* 7:109–19.

Hollander, E. P. 1958. "Conformity, Status, and Idiosyncracy Credit." *Psychological Review* 65:117–27.

Holmes, C. A. 1989. "Health Care and the Quality of Life: A Review." *Journal of Advanced Nursing* 14:833–39.

Hopper, S. 1981. "Diabetes as a Stigmatized Condition: The Case of Low-Income Clinic Patients in the United States." *Social Science and Medicine* 15 B:11–19.

Hyman, M. D. 1971. "Disability and Patients' Perceptions of Preferential Treatment: Some Preliminary Findings." *Journal of Chronic Disease* 24:329–42.

Hyman, M. D. 1972. "Social Isolation and Performance in Rehabilitation." *Journal of Chronic Disease* 28:85–97.

Hyman, M. D. 1975. "Social Psychological Factors Affecting Disability among Ambulatory Patients." *Journal of Chronic Disease* 28:199–216.

Illich, I. 1977. *Medical Nemesis: The Expropriation of Health.* New York: Bantam Books.

Jalowiec, A. 1990. "Issues in Using Multiple Measures of Quality of Life." *Seminars in Oncology Nursing* 6:271–77.

Jennings, B., D. Callahan, and A. L. Caplan. 1988. "Ethical Challenges of Chronic Illness." *Hastings Center Report* 18:S 1–16.

Joint National Committee on the Detection, Evaluation and Treatment of High Blood Pressure. 1984. "The 1984 Report." *Nurse Practitioner* 10:9–33.

Jones, E. E. and K. E. Davis. 1965. "From Acts to Dispositions: The Attributions Process in Person Perception." *Advances in Experimental Social Psychology* 2:219–66.

Jones, E. E., A. Farina, A. H. Hastorf, H. Markus, D. T. Miller, and R. A. Scott. 1984. *Social Stigma: The Psychology of Marked Relationships.* New York: Freeman.

Jones, E. E., and R. E. Nisbett. 1971. *The Actor and the Observer: Divergent Perceptions of the Causes of Behavior.* New York: General Learning Press.

Kalish, R. A. 1977. "Dying and Preparing for Death: A View of Families." In *New Meanings of Death,* ed. H. Feifel. New York: McGraw-Hill.

Kaplan, R. M., S. J. Coons, and J. P. Anderson. 1992. "Quality of Life and Policy Analysis in Arthritis." *Arthritis Care and Research* 5:173–83.

Kasl, S. V., and S. Cobb. 1964. "Some Psychological Factors Associated with Illness Behavior and Selected Illness." *Journal of Chronic Disease* 17:325–45.

Kassenbaum, G., and D. Baumann. 1965. "Dimensions of the Sick Role in Chronic Illness." *Journal of Health and Human Behavior* 6:16–27.

Katz, J. L., H. Weiner, T. F. Gallagher, and I. Hellman. 1970. "Stress, Distress, and Ego Defenses: Psychoendocrine Response to Impending Breast Tumor Biopsy." *Archives of General Psychiatry* 23:131–42.

Katz, S., A. Ford, R. Moskowitz, B. Jackson, and M. Jaffe. 1963. "The Index of ADL: A Standardized Measure of Biological and Psychosocial Function." *Journal of American Medical Association* 185:914–19.

Kelley, H. H. 1967. "Attribution Theory in Social Psychology." In *Nebraska Symposium on Motivation,* ed. D. Levien. Lincoln: University of Nebraska Press.

Kelley, H. H. 1971. *Attribution in Social Interaction.* Morristown, NJ: General Learning Corp.

Kelley, H. H. 1973. "The Process of Causal Attribution." *American Psychology* 28:107–28.

Kemp, B. J., and C. L. Vash. 1971. "Productivity after Injury in a Sample of Spinal Cord Injured Persons: A Pilot Study." *Journal of Chronic Disease* 24:259–75.

Kendall, P., and G. G. Reader. 1979. "Contributions of Sociology to Medicine." In *Handbook of Medical Sociology,* ed. H. E. Greeman, S. Levine, and L. G. Reeder, 1–22. Englewood Cliffs, NJ: Prentice Hall.

Kinchloe, M. 1986. "The Energizing Effect of Purposeful, Creative Activity." *Nursing Forum.* 18:269–77.

Klein, R. F., A. Dean, and M. D. Bogdonoff. 1967. "The Impact of Illness upon the Spouse." *Journal of Chronic Disease* 20:241–48.

Knafl, K. A., and J. A. Deatrick. 1984. "How Families Manage Chronic Conditions: An Analysis of the Concept of Normalization." Paper presented at the Midwest Sociological Association meeting.

Knudson-Cooper, M. S. 1981. "Adjustment to Visible Stigma: The Case of the Severely Burned." *Social Science and Medicine* 15:31–44.

Kobasa, S. C. 1982. "The Hardy Personality: Toward a Social Psychology of Stress and Health." In *Social Psychology of Health and Illness,* ed. G. S. Sanders and J. Sols, 3–32. Hillsdale, NJ: Lawrence Erlbaum.

Koocher, G. P. 1984. "Terminal Care and Survivorship in Pediatric Chronic Illness." *Clinical Psychology Review* 4:571–83.

Krantz, D. S., and A. W. Deckel. 1983. "Coping with Coronary Heart Disease and Stroke." In *Coping with Chronic Disease: Research and Applications,* ed. T. G. Burish and L. A. Bradley. New York: Academic Press.

Krantz, D. S., N. E. Grunberg, and A. Baum. 1985. "Health Psychology." *Annual Review of Psychology* 36:349–93.

Kubler-Ross, E. 1968. *On Death and Dying.* New York: Macmillan.

Langer, E. J., I. L. Janis, and J. A. Wolfer. 1975. "Reduction of Psychological Stress in Surgical Patients." *Journal of Experimental Social Psychology* 11:155–65.

Lau, R. R. 1982. "Origins of Health Locus of Control Beliefs." *Journal of Personality and Social Psychology* 42:322–34.

Lavietes, P. 1974. "The Problem of Chronic Disease." *American Journal of Hospital Pharmacists* 31:1048–52.

Lawrence, R. C., M. C. Hochberg, J. L. Kelsey, F. C. McDuffie, T. A. Medsger, W. R. Felts, and L. E. Schulman. 1989. "Estimates of the Prevalence of Selected Arthritic and Musculoskeleto Diseases in the U.S." *Journal of Rheumatology* 16:327–441.

Lazarus, R. 1966. *Psychological Stress and Coping Process.* New York: McGraw-Hill.

Lazarus, R. 1974. "Psychological Stress and Coping in Adaptation and Illness." *International Journal of Psychiatry in Medicine* 5:321–33.

Lazarus, R. 1982. "Stress and Coping as Factors in Health and Illness." In *Psychological Aspects of Cancer,* ed. J. Cohen, S. W. Cullen, and L. R. Martin, p. 177. New York: Raven Press.

Lazarus, R. 1983. "The Costs and Benefits of Denial." In *The denial of stress,* ed. P. Breznitz, 50–67. New York: International Universities Press.

Lazarus, R., and J. Cohen. 1977. "Environmental Stress." In *Human Behavior and Environment,* vol. 2, ed. I. Altman and J. Wohlwill. New York: Plenum.

Lemert, E. M. 1951. *Social Pathology.* New York: McGraw-Hill.

Lerner, M. J. 1965. "Evaluation of Performance as a Function of Performer's Reward and Attractiveness." *Journal of Personality and Social Psychology* 1:355–60.

Lerner, M. J. 1971. "Observer's Evaluation of a Victim: Justice, Guilt, and Veridical Perception." *Journal of Personality and Social Psychology* 20:127–35.

Lerner, M. J. and G. Matthews. 1967. "Reactions to Suffering of Others under Conditions of Indirect Responsibility." *Journal of Personality and Social Psychology* 5:319–25.

Lerner, M. J., and C. H. Simmons. 1966. "Observer's Reaction to the 'Innocent Victim': Compassion or Rejection?" *Journal of Personality and Social Psychology* 4:203–10.

Levin, L. S., A. H. Katz, and E. Holst. 1979. *Self-Care: Lay Initiatives in Health.* 2d ed. New York: Prodist.

Levine, J. D., and E. Zigler. 1975. "Denial and Self-Image in Stroke, Lung Cancer and Heart Disease Patients." *Journal of Consulting and Clinical Psychology* 43:751–57.

Levine, S., and M. A. Kozloff. 1978. "The Sick-Role: Assessment and Overview." In *Annual Review of Sociology,* ed. R. H. Turner, J. Coleman, and R. Fox, 317–43. Palo Alto: Annual Reviews, Inc.

Lewis, C. E. 1966. "Factors Influencing the Return to Work of Men with Congestive Heart Failure." *Journal of Chronic Disease* 19:1193–1209.

Light, D. 1980. *Becoming Psychiatrists: The Professional Transformation of Self.* New York: Norton.

Light, D. 1990. "The U.S. Health Care System," In *Sociology of Health and Illness,* ed. P. Conrad and R. Kern, 206–14. New York: St. Martin's Press.

Lincoln, Y. S., and E. G. Guba. 1985. *Naturalistic Inquiry.* Beverly Hills, CA: Sage Publications.

Litman, T. J. 1976. *The Sociology of Medicine and Health Care: A Research Bibliography.* San Francisco: Boyd and Fraser.

Locker, David. 1983. *Disability and Disadvantage: The Consequences of Chronic Illness.* London: Tavistock.

Lorber, J. 1967. "Deviance as Performance: The Case of Illness." *Social Problems* 14:302–10.

Lyman, S. M., and M. B. Scott. 1967. "Territoriality: A Neglected Sociological Dimension." *Social Problems* 15:236–49.

MacElveen, P. 1972. "Cooperative Triad in Home Dialysis Care and Patient Outcomes." In *Communicating Nursing Research,* vol. 9, ed. M. Batey. Boulder: WICHEN Publications.

Maddox, G. L., and T. A. Glass. 1989. "Health Care of the Chronically Ill." In *Handbook of Medical Sociology,* 3rd ed., ed. H. Freeman, S. Levine, and L. Reeder. 475–504. Englewood Cliffs, NJ: Prentice Hall.

Markson, E. W. 1971. "Patient Semeiology of a Chronic Disease, Rheumatoid Arthritis." *Social Science and Medicine* 5:159–67.

Markus, H., and E. Wurf. 1990. "The Dynamic Self-Concept: A Social Psychological Perspective." In *Social Psychology Readings: A Century of Research,* ed. A. G. Halberstadt and S. L. Ellyson, 79–88. New York: McGraw-Hill.

Marshall, P. G. 1990. "Setting Limits on Medical Care." *Congressional Quarterly's Editorial Research Reports* no.1:666–78.

McFarlane, A. H., G. R. Norman, D. L. Streiner, and R. G. Roy. 1983. "The Process of Social Stress: Stable, Reciprocal, and Mediating Relationships." *Journal of Health and Social Behavior* 24:160–73.

McKinlay, J. B. 1990. "A Case for Refocussing Upstream: The Political Economy of Illness." In *Sociology of Health and Illness,* ed. P. Conrad and R. Kern, 502–16. New York: St. Martin's Press.

McKinlay, J. B., and S. M. McKinlay. 1990. "Medical Measures and the Decline of Mortality." In *Sociology of Health and Illness,* ed. P. Conrad and R. Kern, 10–23. New York: St. Martin's Press.

Mechanic, D. 1962. "The Concept of Illness Behavior." *Journal of Chronic Disease* 15:189–94.

Mechanic, D. 1972. "Social Psychologic Factors Affecting the Presentation of Bodily Complaints." *New England Journal of Medicine* 286:1132–39.

Mechanic, D. 1974. "Social Structure and Personal Adaptation: Some Neglected Dimensions." In *Coping and Adaptation,* ed. G. Coelho., D. Hamburg, and J. Adams. New York: Basic Books.

Mechanic, D. 1977. "Illness Behavior, Social Adaptation, and the Management of Illness." *Journal of Nervous and Mental Disease* 165:79–87.

Mechanic, D. 1978. *Medical Sociology.* New York: Free Press.

Melvin, J., and S. Nagi. 1970. "Factors in Behavioral Responses to Impairments." *Archives of Physical Medicine and Rehabilitation* 51:552–57.

Meyerowitz., B. E. 1983 "Postmastectomy Coping Strategies and Quality of Life." *Health Psychology* 2:117–32.

Mishel, M. H. 1981. "The Measurement of Uncertainty in Illness." *Nursing Research* 30:258–63.

Mishel, M. H. 1988. "Uncertainty in Illness." *Image: Journal of Nursing Scholarship,* 20:225–32.

Mishel, M. H., T. Hostetter, B. King, and V. Graham. 1984. "Predictors of Psychosocial Adjustment in Patients Newly Diagnosed with Gynecological Cancer." *Cancer Nursing* 7:291–99.

Mishel, M. H., and D. S. Sorenson. 1991. "Uncertainty in Gynecological Cancer: A Test of the Mediating Functions of Mastery and Coping." *Nursing Research* 40:167–71.

Mitchell, G. W., and A. S. Glicksman. 1977. "Cancer Patients: Knowledge and Attitudes." *Cancer* 40:61–66.

Mitteness, L. S. 1987. "So What Do You Expect When You're 85?: Urinary Incontinence in Late Life." In *Research in the Sociology of Health Care: The Experience and Management of Chronic Illness,* vol. 6. ed. Julius A. Roth and Peter Conrad, 177–220. Greenwich, CT: JAI Press.

Moos, R. H. 1964. "Personality Factors Associated with Rheumatoid Arthritis: A Review." *Journal of Chronic Disease* 17:41–55.

Moos, R. H. 1965. "Personality Correlates of the Degree of Functional Incapacity of Patients with Physical Disease." *Journal of Chronic Disease* 18:1019–38.

Moos, R. H. 1976. *The Human Context: Environmental Determinants of Behavior.* New York: Wiley-Interscience.

Moos, R. H., ed. 1977. *Coping with Physical Illness.* New York: Plenum.

Moos, R. H. 1984. "Context and Coping: Toward a Unifying Conceptual Framework." *American Journal of Community Psychology* 12:5–25.

Morrow, G., R. Chiarello, and L. Derogatis. 1978. "A New Scale for Assessing Patients' Psychosocial Adjustment to Medical Illness." *Psychological Medicine* 8:605–10.

Mueller, J. H. 1982. "Self-Awareness and Access to Material Rated as Self-Descriptive or Nondescriptive." *Bulletin of the Psychonomic Society* 19:323–26.

Mullen, B., and J. Suls. 1982. "Know Thyself: Stressful Life Changes and the Ameliorative Effect of Private Self-Consciousness." *Journal of Experimental Social Psychology* 18:43–55.

Mumford, E. 1970. *Interns: From Students to Physicians.* Cambridge, MA: Harvard University Press.

Murdaugh, C. L., and M. H. Mishel. 1991. "Predictors of Quality of Life in Patients Who Undergo Heart Transplantation." Paper presented at the American Heart Association Meeting. Anaheim, CA.

Nadler, A., A. Altman, and J. D. Fisher. 1979. "Helping Is not Enough: Recipients' Reactions to Aid as a Function of Positive and Negative Information about Self." *Journal of Personality* 47:615–28.

National Center for Health Statistics. 1996. *Health, United States, 1995.* Washington, DC: U.S. Government Printing Office.

O'Brien, M. E. 1980. "Effective Social Environment and Hemodialysis Adaptation: A Panel Analysis." *Journal of Health and Social Behavior* 21:360–70.

Oliver, M. J. 1980. "Epilepsy, Crime and Delinquency." *Sociology* 14:417–39.

Parsons, T. 1951. *The Social System.* Glencoe, IL: Free Press.

Parsons, T. 1972. "Definitions of Health and Illness in Light of American Values and Social Structure." In *Patients, Physicians, and Illness,* 2d ed., ed. E. G. Jaco, 120–44. New York: Free Press.

Parsons, T. 1975. "The Sick Role and the Role of the Physician Reconsidered." *Milbank Memorial Fund Quarterly* 53:257–78.

Parsons, T., and R. Fox. 1952. "Illness, Therapy and the Modern Urban American Family." *Journal of Social Issues* 8:31–44.

Pattison, E. M. 1969. "Help in the Dying Process." *Voices* 5:6–14.

Pattison, E. M. 1977. *The Experience of Dying.* New York: Basic Books.

Payer, L. 1988. *Medicine and Culture.* New York: Holt.

Pearlman, R. A., and R. F. Uhlmann. 1988. "Quality of Life in Chronic Diseases: Perceptions of Elderly Patients." *Journal of Gerontology* 43:M25–M30.

Pennebaker, J. W. 1982. *The Psychology of Physical Symptoms.* New York: Springer-Verlag.

Perry, J. A. 1981. "Effectiveness of Teaching in the Rehabilitation of Patients with Chronic Bronchitis and Emphysema." *Nursing Research* 30:219–22.

Population Reference Bureau. 1991. *1991 World Population Data Sheet.* Washington, DC: Population Reference Bureau.

Preston, R. P. 1979. *The Dilemmas of Care: Social and Nursing Adaptations to the Deformed, the Disabled, and the Aged.* New York: Elsevier.

Psathas, G. ed. 1973. *Phenomenological Sociology.* New York: Wiley.

Reif, L. 1975. "Ulcerative Colitis–Strategies for Managing Life." *American Journal of Nursing* 73:261–4.

Relman, A. 1990. "The Trouble with Rationing." *New England Journal of Medicine.* vol 323, 13:911–13.

Richardson, J. L., G. Marks, C. A. Johnson, J. W. Graham, K. K. Chan, J. N. Selser, C. Kishbaugh, Y. Barranday, and A. M. Levine. 1987. "Path Model of Compliance with Cancer Therapy." *Health Psychology* 6:183–207.

Robinson, D. 1971. *The Process of Becoming Ill.* London: Routledge and Kegan Paul.

Rodin, J. 1978. "Somatopsychic and Attribution." *Personality and Social Psychology Bulletin* 4:531–40.

Rodin, M., J. Price, F. Sanchez, and S. McElligot. 1989. "Derogation, Exclusion, and Unfair Treatment of Persons with Social Flaws: Controllability of Stigma and the Attribution of Prejudice." *Personality and Social Psychology Bulletin* 15:439–51.

Roskies, E. 1972. *Abnormality and Normality: The Mothering of Thalidomide Children.* Ithaca, NY: Cornell University Press.

Ross, L. 1977. "The Intuitive Psychologist and His Shortcomings: Distortions in the Attribution Process." In *Advances in Experimental Social Psychology,* ed. L. Berkowitz. New York: Academic Press.

Roth, J. 1963. *Timetables.* Indianapolis: Bobbs-Merrill.

Roth, P., and J. Harrison. 1991. "Orchestrating Social Change: An Imperative in Care of the Chronically Ill." *Journal of Medicine and Philosophy,* 16:343–59.

Rowat, K. M., and K. A. Knafl. 1985. "Living with Chronic Pain: The Spouse's Perspective." *Pain* 23:259–71.

Royer, A. 1995. "Living with Chronic Illness." *Research in the Sociology of Health Care* 12:25–48.

Ryan, W. 1971. *Blaming the Victim.* New York: Pantheon.

Sackett, D. L., and J. C. Snow. 1979. "The Magnitude of Compliance and Noncompliance." In *Compliance in Health Care,* ed. R. B. Haynes, J. C. Taylor, and D. L. Sackett. Baltimore: Johns Hopkins University Press.

Safilios-Rothschild, C. 1970. *The Sociology and Social Psychology of Disability and Rehabilitation.* New York: Random House.

Sarbin, T. R. 1966. *Role Theory: Concepts and Research.* New York: Wiley.

Schachter, S. 1959. *The Psychology of Affiliation.* Stanford, CA: Stanford University Press.

Schatzman, L., and A. L. Strauss. 1973. *Field Research: Strategies for a Natural Sociology.* Englewood Cliffs, NJ: Prentice Hall.

Scheff, T. J. 1966. *Being Mentally Ill.* Chicago: Aldine.

Scheier, M. F., C. S. Carver, and F. X. Gibbons. 1979. "Self-Directed Attention, Awareness of Bodily States and Suggestibility." *Journal of Personality and Social Psychology* 37:1576–88.

Schlenker, B. R. 1980. *Impression Management: The Self-Concept, Social Identity, and Interpersonal Relations.* Belmont, CA: Wadsworth.

Schlenker, B. R. 1985. *The Self and Social Life.* New York: McGraw-Hill.

Schneider, J. and P. Conrad. 1983. *Having Epilepsy: The Experience and Control of Illness.* Philadelphia: Temple University Press.

Schutz, A. 1971. *Collected Papers. Volume I: The Problem of Social Reality.* The Hague: Martinus Nijhoff.

Segall, A. 1976. "The Sick-Role Concept: Understanding Illness Behavior." *Journal of Health and Social Behavior* 17:163–70.

Senate Special Committee on Aging. 1985. Aging in America: Trends and Projections. U.S. Senate Special Committee on Aging and the American Association of Retired Persons, Washington, DC.

Shalit, B. 1977. "Structural Ambiguity and Limits to Coping." *Journal of Human Stress* 3:32–45.

Shaver, K. G. 1970. "Defensive Attribution: Effects of Severity and Relevance on the Responsibility Assigned for an Accident." *Journal of Personality and Social Psychology* 14:101–13.

Short, M., and W. Wilson. 1969. "Roles of Denial in Chronic Hemodialysis." *Archives of General Psychiatry* 20:433–37.

Siegler, M., and H. Osmond. 1979. "The Sick Role Revisited." In *Health, Illness, and Medicine,* ed. Gary Albrecht and Paul C. Higgins, 146–66. Chicago: Rand McNally.

Simmons, R., S. Klein, and R. Simmons. 1977. *The Gift of Life.* New York: Wiley Inter-science.

Singer, E. 1974. "Premature Social Aging: The Social-Psychological Consequences of a Chronic Illness." *Social Science and Medicine* 8:143–51.

Smith, R. 1979. "Disability and the Recovery Process: Role of Social Networks." In *Patients, Physicians, and Illness,* 3d ed., ed. E. G. Jaco. New York: Free Press.

Sontag, S. 1978. *Illness as Metaphor.* New York: Farrar, Straus and Giroux.

Sontag, S. 1989. *AIDS and Its Metaphors.* New York: Farrar, Straus and Giroux.

Starr, P. 1982. *The Social Transformation of American Medicine.* New York: Basic Books.

Stewart, D. C., and T. G. Sullivan. 1982. "Illness Behavior and the Sick Role in Chronic Disease: The Case of Multiple Sclerosis." *Social Science and Medicine* 16:1307–1404.

Stimson, G. V. 1975. "Obeying Doctor's Orders: A View from the Other Side." *Social Science and Medicine* 8:97–104.

Stimson, G. V., and B. Webb. 1975. *Going to See the Doctor: The Consultation Process in General Practice.* London: Routledge and Kegan.

Stone, G. P. and H. A. Farberman. 1970. *Social Psychology Through Symbolic Interaction.* Waltham, MA: Ginn Blaisdell.

Strauss, A. L. 1987. *Qualitative Analysis for Social Scientists.* Cambridge, NY: Cambridge University Press.

Strauss, A. L., and B. Glaser. 1975. *Chronic Illness and the Quality of Life.* Saint Louis: C. V. Mosby.

Strauss, A. L., J. Corbin, S. Fagerhaugh, B. G. Glaser, D. Maines, B. Suczek, and C. L. Wiener. 1984. 2nd. ed. *Chronic Illness and the Quality of Life.* Saint Louis: C. V. Mosby.

Stryker, S. 1980. *Symbolic Interactionalism.* Menlo Park, CA: Benjamin/Cummings.

Suchman, E. A. 1965a. "Social Patterns of Illness and Medical Care." *Journal of Health and Human Behavior* 6:2–16.

Suchman, E. A. 1965b. "Stages of Illness and Medical Care." *Journal of Health and Human Behavior* 6:114–28.

Sudnow, D. 1972. *Studies in Social Interaction.* New York: Free Press.

Syme, L. 1975. "Social and Psychological Risk Factors in Coronary Heart Disease." *Modern Concepts of Cardiovascular Disease* 44:17–21.

Tagliacozzo, D. L., and H. O. Mauksch. 1979. "The Patient's View of the Patient's Role." In *Patients, Physicians, and Illness,* ed. E. G. Jaco, 185–201. New York: Free Press.

Taylor, S. E. 1978. "A Developing Role for Social Psychology in Medicine and Medical Practice." *Personality and Social Psychology Bulletin* 4:515–23.

Taylor, S. E. 1979. "Hospital Patient Behavior: Reactance, Helplessness, or Control?" *Journal of Social Issues* 35:152–58.

Taylor, S. E. 1982. "Social Cognition and Health." *Personality and Social Psychology Bulletin.* 8:549–62.

Taylor, S. E. 1983. "Adjustment to Threatening Events: A Theory of Cognitive Adaptation." *American Psychologist* 38:1161–73.

Taylor, S. E. 1995. *Health Psychology.* 3rd ed. New York: McGraw-Hill.

Taylor, S. E., R. R. Lichtman, and J. V. Wood. 1984. "Attributions, Beliefs about Control, and Adjustment to Breast Cancer." *Journal of Personality and Social Psychology* 46:489–502.

Tessler, R. C., and S. H. Schwartz. 1972. "Help-Seeking, Self-Esteem, and Achievement Motivation: An Attributional Analysis." *Journal of Personality and Social Psychology* 21:318–26.

Twaddle, A. C. 1981. *Sickness Behavior and the Sick Role.* Cambridge, MA: Schenkman.

U.S. Bureau of the Census. 1986. *Statistical Abstract of the United States.* 106th ed. Washington, DC: U.S. Government Printing Office.

U.S. Bureau of the Census. 1987. *Statistical Abstract of the United States.* 107th ed. Washington, DC: U.S. Government Printing Office.

U.S. Department of Health and Human Services (DHHS). Public Health Service. National Center for Health Statistics. 1981. Health, United States. Washington, DC: U.S. Government Printing Office.

U.S. Department of Health, Education and Welfare (DHEW). Public Policy and Chronic Disease. 1979. "A Forum Sponsored by the National Arthritis Advisory Board." Public Health Service Publication No. 79–1896 (May).

Voysey, M. 1972. "Impression Management by Parents with Disabled Children." *Journal of Health and Social Behavior* 13:80–89.

Waddel, C. 1982. "The Process of Neutralization and the Uncertainties of Cystic Fibrosis." *Sociology of Health and Illness* 4:210–20.

Waitzkin, H. 1976. "Information Control and the Micropolitics of Health Care: Summary of an Ongoing Research Project." *Social Science and Medicine.* 10:263–70.

Walster, E. 1966. "Assignment of Responsibility for an Accident." *Journal of Personality and Social Psychology* 3:73–79.

Webster, K. K., and N. J. Christman. 1988. "Perceived Uncertainty and Coping Post Myocardial Infraction." *Western Journal of Nursing Research* 10: 384–400.

West, P. B. 1979a. "An Investigation into the Social Construction and Consequences of the Label Epilepsy." *Sociological Review* 27:719–41.

West, P. B. 1979b."Making Sense of Epilepsy." In *Research in Psychology and Medicine,* ed. D. J. Osborne, M. M. Gruneberg, and J. R. Eiser, 162–69. New York: Academic Press.

Wheeler, L., K. G. Shaver, R. A. Jones, G. R. Goethals, J. Cooper, J. E. Robinson, C. L. Gruder, and K. W. Outzine. 1969. "Factors Determining the Choice of a Comparison Other." *Journal of Experimental Social Psychology* 5:219–32.

Wiener, C. L. 1975. "The Burden of Rheumatoid Arthritis." In *Chronic Illness and the Quality of Life,* ed. A. L. Strauss and B. Glaser, 71–80. St. Louis: C. V. Mosby.

Wineman, N. M. 1990. "Adaptation to Multiple Sclerosis: The Role of Social Support, Functional Disability and Perceived Uncertainty." *Nursing Research* 39:294–99.

Worden, J., and H. Sobel. 1978. "Ego Strength and Psychosocial
    Adaptation   to   Cancer."   *Psychosomatic   Medicine*
    40:585–92.
Zborowski, M. 1952. "Cultural Components in Responses to Pain."
    Journal of Social Issues 8:16–30.
Zborowski, M. 1969. *People in Pain*. San Francisco: Jossey-Bass.
Zola, I. K. 1973. "Pathways to the Doctor – from Person to Patient."
    Social Science and Medicine 7:677–90.
Zola, I. K. 1982. *Missing Pieces: A Chronicle of Living with a
    Disability*. Philadelphia: Temple University Press.
Zola,   I.   K.   1983.   *Socio-Medical   Inquiries: Recollections,
    Reflections,   and   Reconsiderations*.   Philadelphia: Temple
    University Press.
Zola, I. K. 1990. "Helping – Does It Matter: The Problems and
    Prospects of Mutual Aid Groups." Addressed to the United
    Ostomy Association, 1970. In *The Sociology of Health and
    Illness: Critical Perspectives*, ed. P. Conrad and R. Kern,
    502–16. New York: St. Martin's Press.

Index

About the Author

ARIELA ROYER, Assistant Professor of Sociology at Indiana University South Bend, writes and presents conference papers on health and illness issues. She received her Ph.D. from the University of Illinois in 1990. Her primary areas of research are in sociology of health and illness, social psychology, and sociology of mental health.

ISBN 0-275-96123-0

90000>

EAN

9 780275 961237

HARDCOVER BAR CODE